PowerPoint is More than a Slide Program

A Reflective Practice Series

David R Tollafield

Busypencilcase Reflective Communications

Cover by Matt Davies

ISBN:9798667066811

Established 2015

Books by the same author
(available from Amazon)

Podiatry & Foot Health

Clinical Skills in Treating the Foot, Churchill-Livingstone
with Linda Merriman

Assessment of the Lower Limb, Churchill-Livingstone
with Linda Merriman

Morton's Neuroma. Podiatrist Turned Patient: My Own Journey.
A New Foot Pain Series

Bunion. Hallux Valgus. Behind the Scenes.
My Patient Journey Series

Professional Skills

Presenting Your Image
Conferences to Village Halls

Selling Foot Health as Podiatry
Communication, Promotion and Branding

Children

The Story of Cristal Rouge
(as Rob C Blyth)

'The important part of speaking is to sound natural and as if you were having a cosy chat. This means you must know what you want to say but should not try to learn what you need to say.' Author

All illustrations used in this book are licensed from Shutterstock^{TM} unless stated other materials are my own.

The PowerPoint screen pictures are called screen captures and have been modified to show the specific icons and working of slide compilation based on version 15.18 (C) 2015

Table of Contents

Acknowledgements

Most books have an acknowledgement page for a good reason; while this work is mine, my beta readers have allowed me to beat through the thick scrubland that emerged over the two years to produce two books on speaking in public.

Thanks to Roy Jones who provided inspiration and encouragement and Simon Whitfield, Director at Profile Productions. I continue to enjoy working with your very professional crew with the joys of making PowerPoint work at conferences. My thanks also go to Associate Professor Reza Naraghi in Australia for having the confidence to recognise the book's potential for students and importantly to Professor David Pratt who suggested this book as a companion. I am also grateful to Mr Ian Reilly who made time to read my first draft.

I would like to credit Joanna Penn, Eric Bergman and Chris Davidson who made me think outside the box and to Akash Karia who confirmed many of my ideas when designing image based slides. I am grateful to Matt Davies who stepped in at short notice to design the cover, and, finally, to audiences and future readers for listening to me and purchasing this book; may it bring you luck, confidence and direction.

No personal or financial inducement was made in the production of this book

Preface

'PowerPoint is More than a Slide Program' is not intended as the ultimate PowerPoint Manual but inevitably there is some resemblance. It is an introductory resource for the wannabe speaker, but I hope this book provides inspiration in how to build a talk with PowerPoint in mind. If you have never used PowerPoint before, these pages will offer you a guide in designing your slide deck for your talk and highlight some of the do's and don'ts from the start.

You can buy PowerPoint for Dummies, Google a specific question or look up YouTube for anything that you are unsure about, but, remember your comfort zone will come with practice and the technology will feel less daunting.

It is useful to appreciate that while PowerPoint has a large range of options, you will probably only require a small number of the features mentioned in these pages. However, animations and transitions, colour and text can enhance your talk if used well, but sadly this is often not the case. The version of PowerPoint used in this book may well be known to many, but newer versions exist as there is constant development. While references and illustrations relate only to this version, the principles remain the same.

I learnt to use PowerPoint the hard way and made many mistakes. No-one showed me how to use this package or the pitfalls associated with PowerPoint but typically I followed others, and of course, embraced their mistakes.

IF you like PowerPoint when designing talks, then this book is for you. If you are a novice, then definitely YES. IF you are experienced but feel your presentations are not top form, YES this book actually tries to tear you away from some of the problems that may have crept in with your designs. Remember the better you think that you are, the harder it is to reflect on bad habits. I am a huge fan of PowerPoint but realised that I had used PowerPoint badly. The sections have been set out as chapters, many are short and succinct and allow you to dip in and out depending upon your prior knowledge.

This book is a companion to ***Projecting Your Image*** which covers the rules of how to speak in public with PowerPoint in mind, the latter without the technical detail. Having written the first book, I wanted to put in more examples of how to build a talk and to provide more detail about using PowerPoint, so here it is. A companion book should support, fill in missing details and also provide some sense of application where other books cannot travel. I have tried to avoid overlap but there will be the occasional cross over that I hope provides a good link between both books and offers a different perspective. As I often give talks on public speaking, these books naturally become a source for those who attend. Please follow my website for more information on talks. It might seem strange but it is www.consultingfootpain.co.uk

If you have enjoyed this book or want to add any comments, please do contact me by davidt@busypencilcase.com. Your Amazon review would be most welcome.

David R Tollafield

Part 1
Background

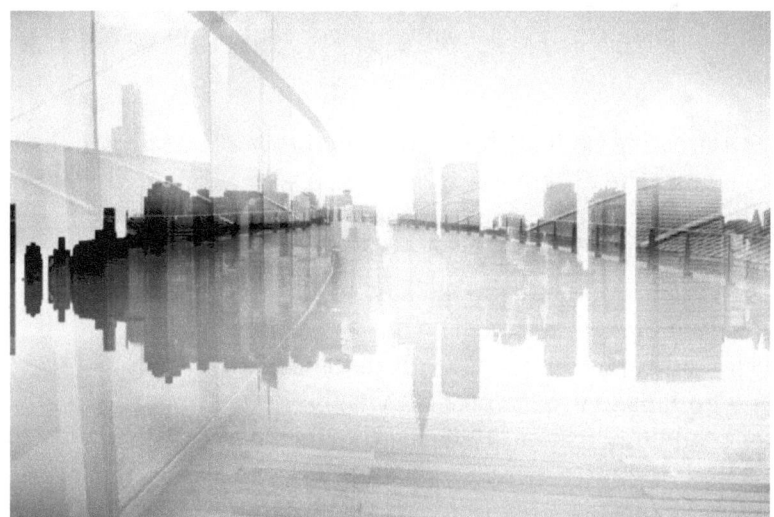

© Rawpixel

A GENERAL OVERVIEW

1 - Justifying PowerPoint

Without doubt there are detractors who are not in favour of using PowerPoint when speaking. I am not one of them but I am aware of the dangers of poor design. However, there is much wisdom in those critics that say that reliance on PowerPoint can create an adverse effect on your audience, including sending them to sleep. Boredom leads to poor audience reviews and material that might be of value is diminished.

There is a growing body of speakers who throw a slide deck together to make a talk. The difference in quality between such presentations is palpable and has vexed some to speak out about using PowerPoint badly. Examples of critics are cited within these pages and referenced at the end of the book. This in some ways has led to condemnation of PowerPoint. The makers of PowerPoint only provide a facility. It is not Microsoft that make a talk poor but the speaker who fails to use the product wisely. PowerPoint represents modern technology that has replaced the blackboard. There will be a new generation shortly that will have never known what chalk and talk was about outside Victorian School Museums.

PowerPoint has not just replaced the blackboard though, but the overheard projector (OHP) and the 35 mm slide projector, and for good reasons. Digital images are easier to produce because the system offers more flexibility.

However, where there is a poor relationship between the speaker's words or oratory, the use of text on the slide can subsume audience concentration. While you might feel using visual technology is about being a technical geek, it isn't. Writing acetates for the OHP meant wads of transparencies (called acetates) building up. They would deteriorate in time, or have to be updated. Preparation time and mistakes were harder to correct. PowerPoint offered a new method whereby fast editing and design was possible.

Thirty-five millimetre slides on the other hand were expensive to produce if you wanted text. The process was lengthy and slides had to be photographed with expensive equipment and then turned into transparencies. Again PowerPoint offered a new way forward allowing text to be created with exciting colours, designs and backgrounds.

Flexibility and compactness

PowerPoint does not just fill a niche, it has revolutionised everything about public speaking. A slide presentation can be condensed and stored onto a portable file using a Universal Serial Bus (USB) memory stick also called a flash drive. The file can be sent by e-mail and downloaded at another location. All those transparencies and slides previously can now be given a professional feel and brand users offered a valuable method to promote their message and product.

Slides can be manipulated so they could be moved around in different order and images previously static can be made dynamic with embedded video clips. It is not hard then to realise for reasons of portability, storage, editing, reduced cost and convenience, the process behind public speaking has changed for good.

Other digital programmes

PowerPoint is not the only digital slide system. Others exist and a large number of alternatives offer similar options to PowerPoint, some from a different perspective. Keynote and Prezi have now been joined by Visme, Haiku Duck and Emaze. These additional software programmes are by no means the only programmes, but the object of this book is not to go into each one, as more material can be found on the internet in greater detail.

Designing a slide, compiling text, acquiring quality pictures, importing and problems with data size will consume the speaker when first introduced to PowerPoint as delving into multiple systems serves little purpose.

Getting stuck in

I first experimented with PowerPoint in 1996 and acquired new upgrades every time I changed my laptop or desktop. I made many mistakes of which the biggest was to use every feature that I could. Today I try to create a basic format and keep it clean and simple.

In this book I have set out to explain how images in PowerPoint can be built around a certain economy to benefit the audience. Of course if we have to put writing with any slide remember that PowerPoint does not deliver the talk alone it required voice and image. To design a PowerPoint slide deck with all the facilities available is asking for a number of disasters. I have emphasised against creating a slide deck for the sake of using visual imagery - just because you create an image on a slide is not the same as producing the image you need.

Having made my own mistakes and cited authors such as Chris Davidson and Eric Bergman, two passionate speakers who advise against PowerPoint in different ways, I have tried to balance the arguments objectively.

Slide presentations are here to stay and if done well will enhance the talk and lecture experience. Packed with gismos and with off the shelf options, you can erroneously spin a whirlwind creation that steals from your talk.

We are all novices[1] at some point and try to emulate others who we respect. There is nothing at fault with this philosophy but the difference between an experienced speaker and a novice is like trying to swim the English Channel after only completing your 25 metres certificate. Some speakers may undertake regular talks on a circuit, and will have presented for years. Their easy style is drawn from dogged hours of preparation marinated in the experience of performing for many years.

The Ground Rules

I have borrowed a little from my book, '*Projecting Your Image*'. Those expected to give a conference talk may find some assistance in knowing that there are ground rules that can guide and improve technique whilst instilling confidence. Your talk boils down to following a few rules and if unbroken, will ensure your talk or presentation runs smoothly.

Packing a subject into a short period of engagement becomes the first obstacle. What to keep in? What to leave out? Avoiding being too superficial or risking overshooting. These are just some of the concerns novices will experience.

If we consider our slides as a 'deck of cards', we suddenly find it all too easy to overpopulate the talk and spend a disproportionate time on *IMAGES* rather than develop the narrative.
To compensate for time lost, those spoken words are placed as chunks of sentences onto our slides. This act can raise the veiled hope that the audience will read what we might not have said and therefore save time on our delivery. This does not work!

---

[1] 'The Novice'. Someone who lacks experience or seeks a new skill.

One of your next obstacles to overcome is fear, stage fright and those so called nerves. The fear of adverse judgement, forgetting to say something you later regret omitting, is only part of the scenario. Letting down colleagues can lay heavily on your subconscious state.

As the day draws ever closer toward your debut you now sew doubts about your ability. From your perspective when all seems fine and the talk should hang together, your brain stops functioning and the words fail to come out. Then, confronted with anxiety about performing well, you have a remote control for your slide programme in one hand. If a slide accidently fast forwards several slots, your presentation sequence is knocked off course. You glance up at the screen and panic as your try to reverse the slide.

Memory and learning

You do not need to learn your talk by heart, just know where you need to add narrative. This also means knowing when to stop and not over-talk. And so the more work you put into your preparation the result will be more visible and pleasing because it will look effortless.

Location & effect

It might seem that a talk given at a conference or large meeting is more important than at a village hall. However, professional reputations can be made or lost especially if the talks are for financial or reputational reward or business.

Local group meetings might mean you don't get invited back as word gets around. When not for reward, but pleasure, you might be a little more relaxed.

I find conference meetings more intimidating as one is competing with other speakers in the same field. Casual meetings are more fun as there is less scrutiny about content.

Preparation time

I spend more time than some, less than others when preparing. I may not be efficient as I like to cruise a little, reading around my subject, and play with diagrams and drawings. I am a slide geek but equally feel my talks do better with images. However, we don't want to achieve the expression; *Death by PowerPoint!*

If you know a subject particularly well you probably are able to stand up and talk off the cuff. Making a few notes to keep order and select slides to fit the talk will not take long. This is the position you would want to be if you intended doing a fair amount of public speaking. Once a talk has been delivered, refined and repeated, the effort reduces. If you have never ever talked in public and have never presented at a conference, then you are a novice.
Speaking provides confidence to your personality and allows you to project your own image and help to sell your skills for financial gain or career development, or simply support continuous professional development skills. Continuous professional development is about updating your knowledge.

Any role that requires close contact with the public (clients, patients, users and providers) will depend on good communication. Awareness of spoken language and clarity is important as well as learning about timing.

We can now assume two things in regard to the novice. You want to speak or need to speak and are willing to have a crack at it. I have included a few tips and guides here, but more detail can be found in my book; *Projecting Your Image.*

Familiar specialist topic

If motivated by your subject, you will already have a good deal of information. Your task will be to put it in the right order, but know what to leave in and take out. However, we cannot reproduce all that we know in a short period. You must aim to consider what message you want to convey and no more as this forms the **Purpose** of our talk. If undertaking the task as a solo speaker use your question and answer time (Q&A) to expand, not during the talk. Do not become complacent because you know your subject matter. Timing, pace, and use of the right words will still require practise.

Unfamiliar content

Undertake a trial run. Take a section of your proposed talk. It does not have to be refined at this point. Select a close friend or partner or someone you that know who will not mind providing feedback. Write out some prompt (cue) cards to keep yourself in the correct order. Make sure your head comes up to project your voice above the cards. Try to speak slowly even if this seems odd. If you do not want to use someone to listen to you consider recording your voice.

Making the title interesting

Naturally any title you select will depend on your own point of view and what you personally find interesting. Take a talk about the *Channel Island of Jersey*. Because the island has Anglo-French links this will broaden the subject and could lead to an enormous amount of material being generated. You can always leave finishing off the title until your content has been worked out. However, groups and conference organisers will prefer a title in advance of their programme so do give the title serious thought.

Content and target

Build the content using research material needed for the talk. You cannot import research directly into content, it will need reassembling. You will have to trim a good deal away. Find the elements of the story and if possible an angle that can hook the audience. A story board will help you retain some focus, but it is very easy to allow images to run away at this stage (chapter 8). Think of a bullseye target. The centre is your lecture honed to perfection. The outer rings are the early material while the outermost ring is your 'raw' research. The target analogy relates to the ever decreasing diameter of the coloured circles as each ring becomes smaller toward the centre. The finite sized bullseye area relates to the main purpose of your talk, honed with brevity in mind.

Research

This feature is where most of your preparation will come from. Pound to a penny you will hit Google and any home reference books you have on your shelf. Old brochures might be useful or maybe take a trip to the library and do some photocopying. Keep those holiday snaps of Jersey handy but do not start using them yet because if you do you will create too many.

'I must use that one, and then yes, I must use this one...'

Don't feel ashamed we have all attested to similar temptations.

Resources in general

Here are some more resources. *National Trust* second hand book shops make great places to browse. National Trust are inexpensive because you can pick up books from 50p - £2.00 without postage[2]. Second hand book shops are more expensive than the National Trust but they are run as a going concern and books have to be purchased while National Trusts books are donated.

Amazon allows
    a) a search by author and title
    b) offers second hand and new books which
    may be as cheap as 0.01p, then you need to
    pay postage.

If the subject is more technical and you need to use a library for academic support, then you will have to pay for any searches. A search is carried out by professional librarian on your behalf. The *British Lending Library* in Boston (UK) and London houses past publications. This is a big area to explain in detail but professionals who study academic subjects have a head start especially if associated with an academic institution. On-line access is now very much in vogue and a professional journal or websites with back articles can be useful, especially if there is a relationship with an academic institution. Because more journals are electronically published you can download them from the publisher's website. If a journal has a digital objective identifier code (DOI) you can use the code from anywhere and place it into your finder space on your search engine and the journal will download.

https://doi.org/10.1186/s13047-017-0225-2[3].

---

[2] Applicable to 2019.The visitor is often invited to drop money into an honesty box. The money helps the National Trust so don't abuse this privilege please.

[3] HTTPS stands for Hypertext Transfer Protocol Secure

You do not need the 'https' before the dot but you must ensure the remaining code is accurate. Doi.org/10.1186/s13047-017-0225-2 *Abe books* in the USA carry books out of print at a reasonable price. Do not forget the use of newspapers as a resource. These can help create the mood of a period in time. Upon locating a source go to the references and bibliography section where more material might be quoted to fit the need of your content. It is easy to see why all of this takes time and you may think it not worth it. Work put in produces effect out and a good effect is required if you believe in pride.

Consider these questions.

> How much research do you need to provide content, or varied content?
> What is your time-line to carry out research?
> What is your budget?

Once you have your raw material extract passages of relevant information and make notes as you go. Don't expect to remember where you found information at the end when you have a stack of reference material. This stack becomes your resource file. When I was at University we were taught to use blank postcards available from stationers. This is a great tool because you can enter headings on a card, then indicate where to find each source. Add in a brief summary about content and now you have a method of moving material around to fit into your talk. You can use your PC or laptop but sometimes hard copy is safer. Research is my favourite part of planning as I learn so much. The volume can be daunting as your material can grow at an alarming rate. By-pass research and your talk will diminish in its potential 'grab value'. Aim for depth. You can always shed material, but, equally do not cram it all into your lecture or you will cause audience overload. You can guess. I have done this and yes regretted it.

Other forms of visual aid

While majority of this book is biased toward speaking with the assistance of PowerPoint and slide images, for smaller group presentations other methods can be used that have less technical involvement. It is worth mentioning these as well as CCTV (closed circuit television) methods.

CCTV is useful for demonstration to large groups and if models are used or practical techniques such as preparation of cooking, this allows the detail to be seen. In fact, big conferences today use CCTV links projected onto large screens so every crease and fold of a speakers' face is visible.

Paper flip-charts or white boards are helpful for small groups, being of value for longer interactive sessions based on a work shop style[4]. The use of black boards has little place in most speaking situations outside of formal teaching. In many cases such methods have been surpassed by digital white boards.

For some years I used acetate sheets. You can draw on these with coloured inked pens and the image is projected against any white surface. Newer projectors can collapse and store better. Some acetate sheets can be copied onto the acetate in colour or black and white. Prepared before a talk these carry as much value as PowerPoint slides. Finding an overhead projector (OHP) is not so easy today in many venues but they still have a place and are available.

It is important to decide if your talk requires audio-visual assistance and whether technical support is needed. The laptop and projector is very utilitarian and slide programmes can be mailed out ahead of the talk in a format that can be compressed or *Zip filed*. The images can also be saved in different formats.

---

[4] **Workshops.** While a speaker will talk at such events there is usually more interaction from the audience participating in exercises. Formal talks are limited in this scenario.

2 - Jabber rabbit

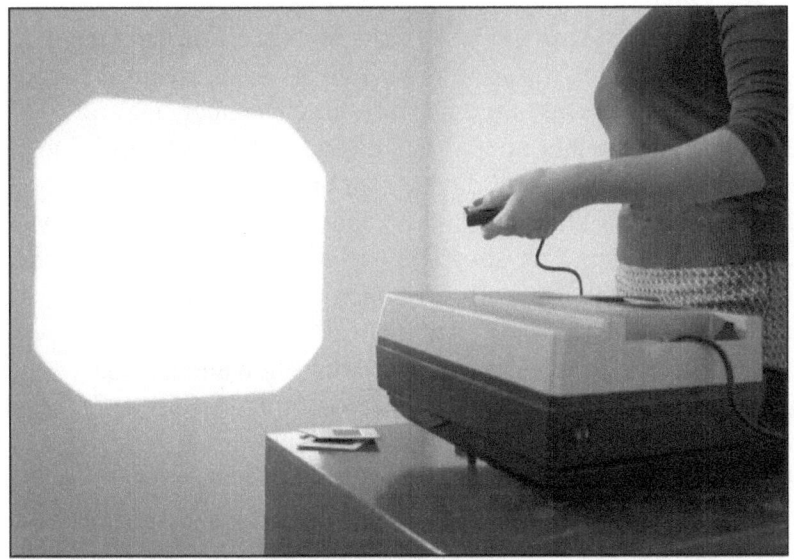

'BUT HOW WAS I TO KNOW YOU'D BEND MY EARHOLES TOO?
WITH YOUR INCESSANT TALKIN',
YOU'RE BECOMING A PEST,'

LYRICS: CHAS HODGES & DAVE PEACOCK

Length of Talk[5]

---

[5] © THPStock - old style slide projector. This offered less flexibility with text slides which once produced were permanent.

As speakers we will use our subject matter to draw people. If we are known, or indeed have written on the subject, this may attract an audience effectively to our talk. We ideally want to draw people to us because we speak effectively. For some, the art of speaking comes naturally, but it will depend on the occasion.

Henry V made his famous battle cry speech before Agincourt during the 100 year's war between England and France. Abraham Lincoln provide a historical speech at Gettysburg. Winston Churchill gave rousing speeches during the second world war. All these might come to mind for their powerful effect because they were concise and resonated with human emotions. Then of course there was the Cuban Leader, Fidel Castro, who could speak for hours, probably as he thought that was the right thing to do. What might come to mind was the fact that he was unaware someone had to listen to him. Rarely do we find public speeches do well when they are about the person speaking, or where they ramble with little direction.

Initially we want to design a talk that has direction and secondly, where slide image has value, create an instant memorable relationship with the spoken word (oratory). Our aim is to design a method using images or text to enhance but does not distract our talk.

A one-off or a professional role?

Leaving aside those who could or can rise to the occasion, for most of us, public speaking is a one off, often created by necessity. School teachers and university lecturers are a group on their own so are left out of this discussion. This does not mean that teachers and lecturers cannot improve as anyone who offers such a skill should constantly evaluate his or her effectiveness. Our talk will comprise content, delivery and integrate imagery to support our content.

When I first decided to write about speaking in public I was drawn to my own experience with using PowerPoint. Having looked closely at people I respected, I saw flaws even with experienced colleagues. Many used slides which were often redundant, had little value, and more importantly were a source of jabber, or wasted effort. I used 35 mm transparencies and overhead projectors prior to digital projectors with some talk and chalk on a standard blackboard. After teaching for 10 years I pounced on digital slides with relish. Above all they saved time, offered creativity and better marketing. I have experimented with most components of PowerPoint between acquiring new versions. To design a PowerPoint slide deck alone with all the facilities available is asking for a number of disasters, more so if you create slides for the sake of picture placement. I will repeat this emphasis a few times against creating a slide deck for the sake of using visual imagery in order to thump home the message.

T.E.D Talks

Because of the short span of audience concentration, a new breed of talk called the **TED talk** observes a rule to talk for no longer than 18 minutes. TED stands for *technology, entertainment and design* and came about in 1984 being conceived by Richard Wurman in the USA.

Greta Thunberg, the teenager who brought global warming into focus at the age of 15 was respected for her passionate and punchy presentation. She used a TED talk without slides. The talk went viral using a single theme. Her message was clear – *the environment is being ruined for the next generation. Don't leave it later to do something, do it now!* Many other well know orators use TED talks to convey similarly strong messages.

3 - Getting started

Tell that story well

Your objective is to tell a story, capture your audience and engage with them. Your audience needs to buy into your talk without image overload. Images as pictures alone can be forgiven, but text slide overload is a disease which has affected many otherwise good speakers. However, the combination of talk and use of imagery is critical to good presenting. You can go without images, but in our modern world imagery is important. Remember the original Asian saying;

'Hearing something a hundred times isn't better than seeing it once.'
This turned into *'a picture paints a thousand words.'*

Two for the price of One

Story Board:

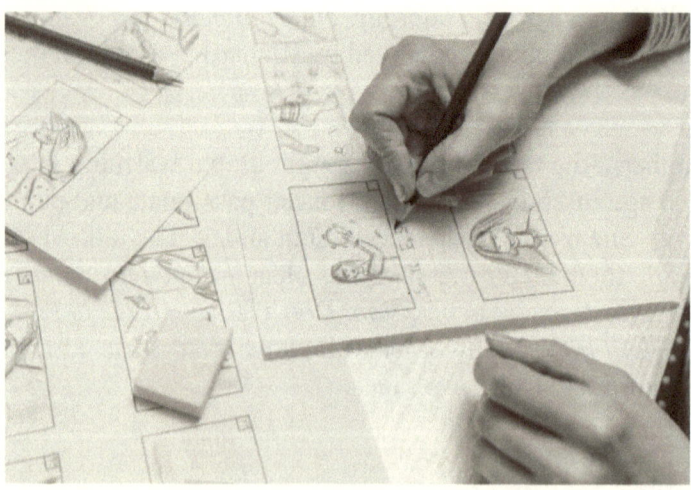

You sit down at your computer and there is a strong temptation to set up those slides first. But here is an important fact. You can still use tools like PowerPoint to plan a talk even if you decide not to use the programme. Let's assume we are going to plan our talk using PowerPoint. This is akin to a film director using a series of *story boards*[6] set out with a start-middle-end scenario. Few authors talk about using PowerPoint as a story board. While the story board will be dealt with here, the remaining book covers the overall objective of facilitating good imagery for text and picture images.

Content images:

To differentiate the second function, projecting your image, this will be covered with a view to creating the content for talking (oratory). You need a **purpose** for the talk so what is your message? Can this be given with the aid of imagery and how much discussion is required. Your **performance** will depend how your images marry to your talk.

---

[6] © Sasha. The story in words rather than pictures.

Part 2
Building with PowerPoint

© Sergiy Kuzmin

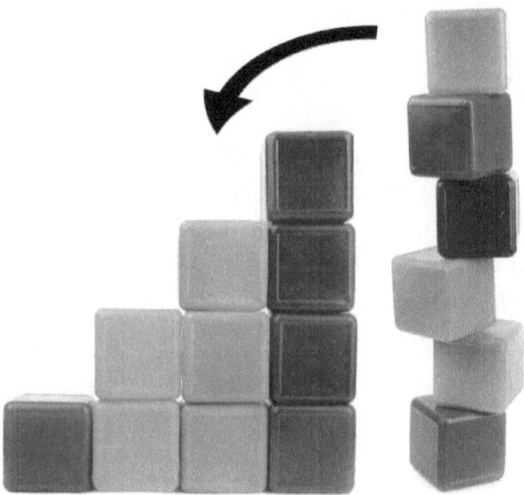

ORGANISED BUILDING IS REQUIRED BEFORE WE STAND AND SPEAK

It is worth remembering building involves using the right slide for the job. A header slide, content, appropriate images and text. What you start with you will certainly not finish with after editing. Building will continue until your talk is tested, edited and honed.

4 - PowerPoint the Planner

Backing up your data

'Autobackup'[7] should be on automatically but make sure the work is saved either to the hard drive which exists within the computer, or a use a *Cloud* type backup (accessible from any computer).

There are a number of different systems that allow data to be stored on a Cloud. Here is a definition from Google, one of the mainstay search engines. Once you increase the data stored on free access systems, and don't forget images are a form of data and take up a great deal of room, then you will need to purchase extra space. If you keep data on your own computer, such storage can slow down the working speed.

What exactly is the cloud?
In the simplest terms, **cloud** computing means storing and accessing data and programs over the Internet instead of your computer's hard drive. The **cloud** is just a metaphor for the Internet. ... The **cloud** is also not about having a dedicated network attached storage (NAS) hardware or server in residence

---

[7] Autobackup is pre-set but can fail so be aware. Usually a message will show on your screen to make you aware Autobackup is not functioning.

Storage systems

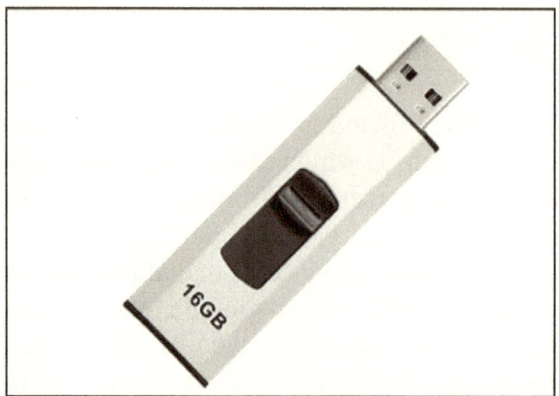

Memory stick/free picture product

Dropbox or similar capacity storage like Cloud[8] means that you can access your work from other locations and devices. There are plenty of examples. A USB (universal serial bus) flash drive or external driver are important utilities to save work. The USB part is simply the shape of the end like a plug that goes into a slot in the computer called a PORT. So we talk about USB ports and USB flash drives. The stick shown, also known as a *memory stick* has 16GB or gigabytes written on the side. This informs the purchaser of the maximum data that can be stored on the device. An external drive is a hard disk that connects to the computer and is free standing (see chapter 23). The advantage of the external drive is that it is small and therefore portable, but has the capacity for holding larger amounts of data, measured in terabytes. This means that there is a great deal more capacity available on external hardware. Don't store slide programmes on any storage that cannot hold the data comfortably. Memory sticks can become corrupted and fail and it is better to purchase well known brand names than cheaper copies. A section on transferring data is considered in chapter 23.

[8]https://www.which.co.uk/reviews/antivirus-software-packages/article/how-to-choose-the-best-cloud-storage-service

5 - Creating a New File for PowerPoint

Everyone is keen to get going. If you know all this stuff and it is too basic, then skip to the next section or use the content to guide you to the parts you want. Again don't forget that newer and older packages of PowerPoint are different and it is the how to improve your slide construction rather than how to use PowerPoint that is the main focus.

Once you have opened PowerPoint, click onto **'New'**. Creating a file as in Word or Excel keeps all your material in one place. Files are often called **documents** as opposed to the term **folders** and contain your slides. Folders are used to contain the documents or files in an ordered place for retrieval. I will use the term files for documents in this book. Initially you will need to open up a slide programme. Select one of the boxes in the illustration, also called panes.

Tip: I would suggest selecting the top left pane, the **blank presentation** as your first option as a novice.

Creating a file is different from creating a new slide. Assign a memorable name to your file, call it Version 1.0 (or V.10 for short).

A date within the file name is useful so you can always distinguish updates. The picture over the page illustrates opening up a new file and the choice of slide images that the user is presented with (with the block arrow).

Overall picture of the first screen shot[9]

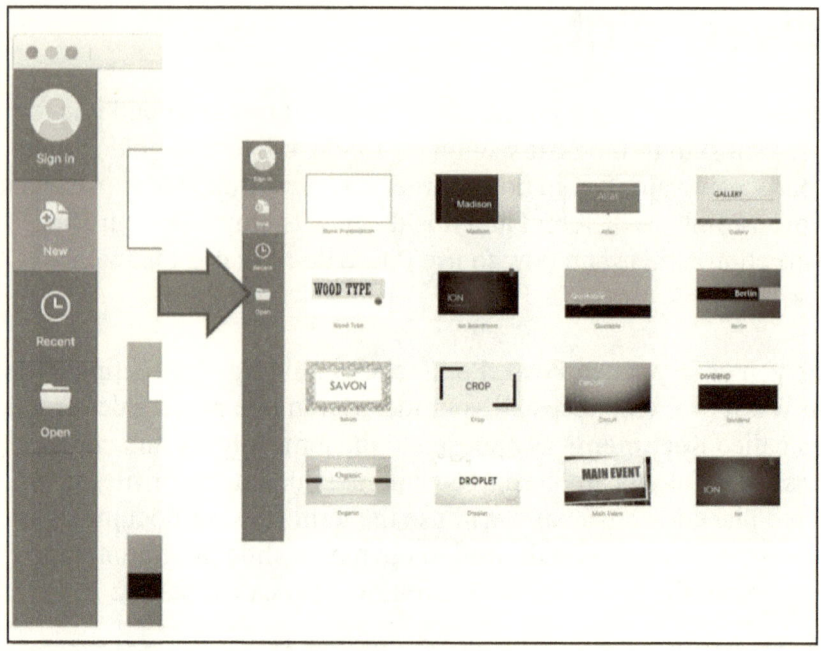

Please note: Further information concerning backing up and saving is dealt with in chapter 23

Select **'File'** on the top horizontal bar next to PowerPoint, then **'save as'.**
Assign your file a name.

This type of presentation is called .pptx which means the file will have a suffice .pptx. PPTX is the stem for PowerPoint instead of .docx as in Word.

---

[9] A larger version of this illustration can be found in Chapter 6

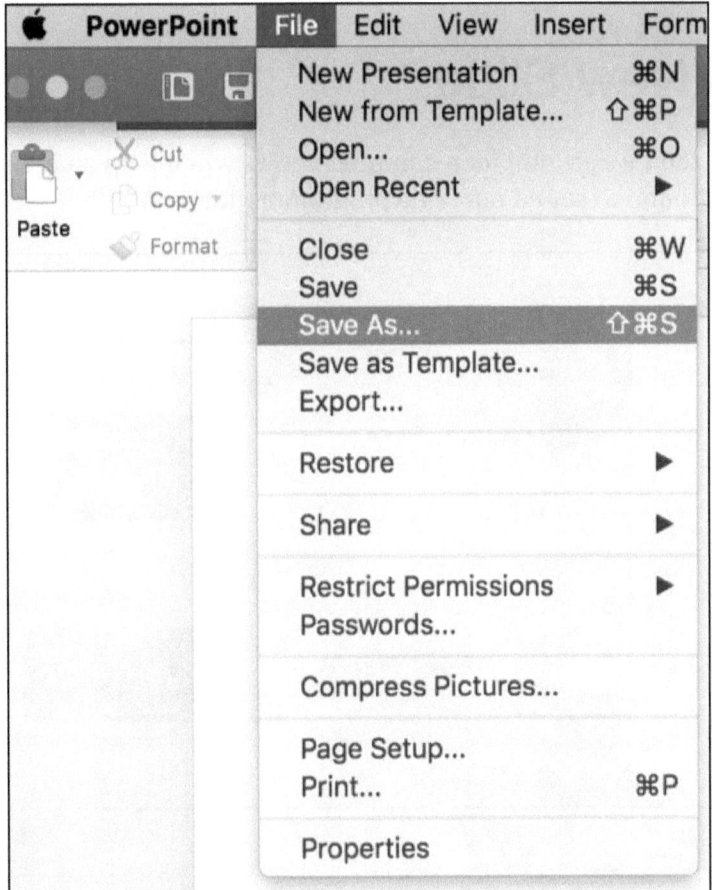

I have called it 'My New talk' and saved it under 'where' i.e the destination called to Desktop - iCloud (see below). You can send the file to any destination on your computer.

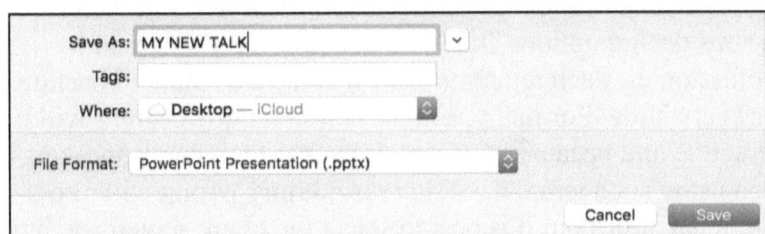

6 - New Slide

Click the PowerPoint icon coloured with a white P on an orange background to set up our slide programme for your talk.

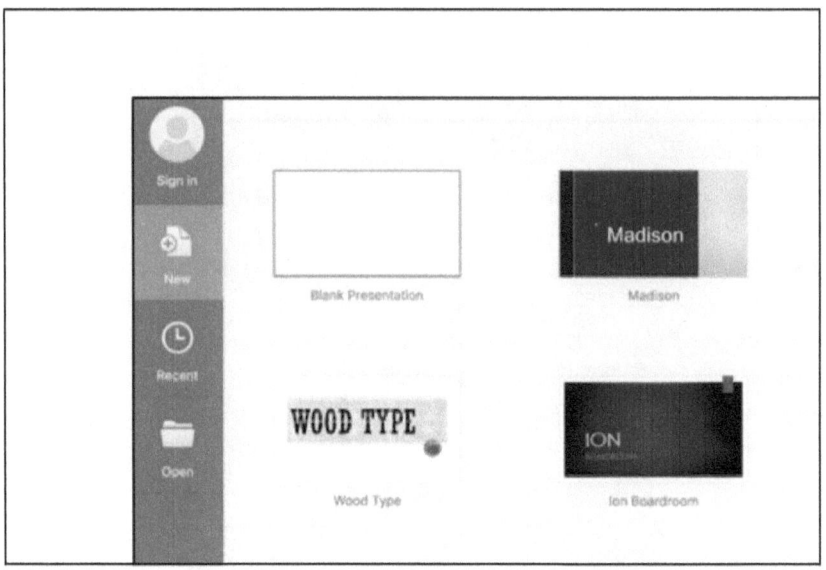

The screen above will appear depending upon the version you are using.

Custom versus template

The image panes (boxes) will offer you an embedded background or template. Colours and patterns, lines and circles will blend with various design options and of course look very smart and professional. Each template used will have a standard background for every slide. For many, some of these unique designs will be attractive and because of the professional feel, many speakers can be seen using such templates. There is nothing wrong with pre-formatted slides but it is best to select the blank screen and build your own slide. This offers more flexibility when you want to change.

Blank slide template (custom)

The reason to suggest using a blank presentation slide is that your own images ideally will consume most if not all of the screen, blocking out the pre-formatted slide. Secondly you can establish your own colour scheme and avoid complex patterns confusing your audience during your talk.

The former 35mm slide was replaced by the digital slide -

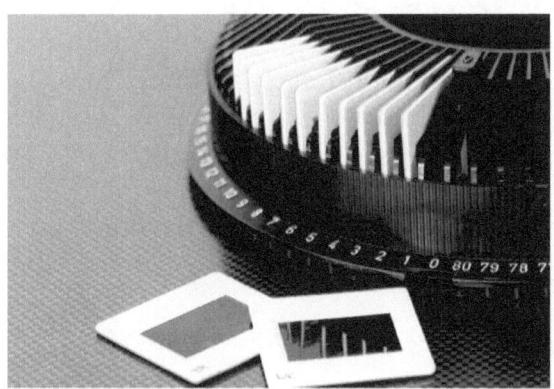

this was the colour transparency slide we used, but less frequently now, although you will still see some using this older technology. The picture is adjusted by the projector lens zooming out to use the full screen space (see the illustration at the start of chapter 2).

When using PowerPoint, and certainly the later versions, the width of the projected image has increased and appears more rectangular in shape. The main aim of the image is to take as much space up, appear clear and large so all can see the detail (refer also to page 63).

7 - Selecting from the PowerPoint information bar

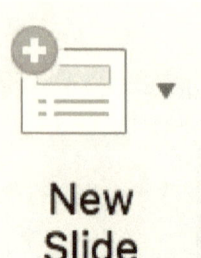

New Slide

The bar below is typical of the PowerPoint software programme and will be repeated again in this book. Forming a new slide can be made after your file has been created and saved. DO back up early and regularly. The information bar provides diagrams and icons (pictorial labels) for different functions. Once you have created a new slide programme save this as a file which you will name for ease of location later on. It is important to make a copy or back-up.

Starting from left to right and represented by the titles below.

Home
Insert
Design
Transitions
Animations
Slide Show
Review
View

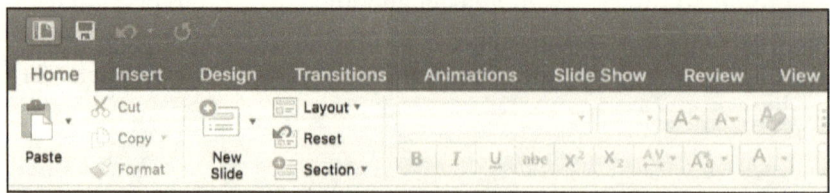

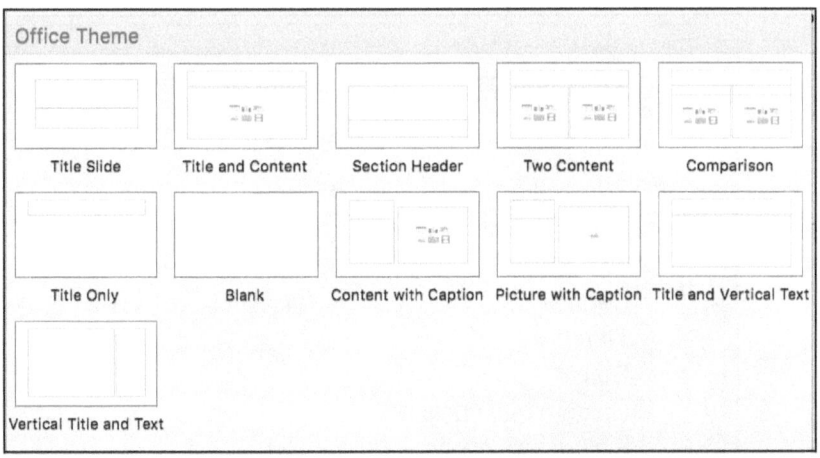

The icon for NEW SLIDE, shown at the top of the last page can be identified under **'Design'**. This is selected and activated by *clicking on*, and by double tapping the mouse.

The first thing you will have to select is the type of slide theme called **Office Theme**, as part of a package that PowerPoint uses called 'Office'. Office also includes Word and Excel packages[10] as well as PowerPoint.

Options

If you select the blank presentation you will find another box that will be offered for further selection with *eleven options* as shown above. The illustration has been summarised as a text box where the bold type indicates the most useful options over the page.

---

[10] **Word** is a word processor system and **Excel** a spreadsheet system under the brand Microsoft.

Office theme

Title slide
Title and content
Section header
Two content
Comparison
Title only
Blank
Content with caption
Picture with caption
Title and vertical text
Vertical title and Text

Office Theme. Slide template[11] designs available.

One thing you will find is that there is more than one way to achieve the endgame. Icons[12] within the various templates offer broad options. The slide with these icons provides another route to adding more features.

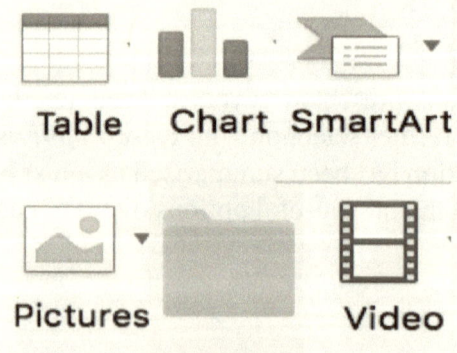

Table   Chart   SmartArt

Pictures   Video

---

[11] **Templates** are taken to mean a pre-set arrangement as opposed to a blank template you build yourself.
[12] **Icons** are picture and diagrams that express a function when actively clicked. A double click or tap might be required on the mouse or finger pad.

The scenario in the slide on page 36 shows six icons in the centre of a pre-set slide. The top left icon represents a **table**, comprising columns and rows. The middle top icon marked **chart**, depicts graphs, while the top right promotes **SmartArt** features. SmartArt provides shapes and designs that might appeal in setting out elements of your talk as boxes, arrows, circles and other interesting shapes (Chapter 21, basic artwork). The bottom left icon, or **Pictures,** is a direct way of importing an image from somewhere else. This could be from your own photo album or from a stock library. The bottom middle icon is a file that contains **text** or other materials, and lastly, **video.** A film can be imported to provide moving images. The term embedding a video feature (in a slide) is often used. Video that requires the internet to run a downloadable film such as a YouTube video is more unpredictable than video that stands alone from an existing file within your own computer storage. Video may be made by the speaker using his or her own digital camera and is usually stored as a file without need for the internet. In order not to complicate matters I will not discuss the use of video further as these are dynamic images that can become troublesome even in expert hands.

Understanding the icons and titles

As a novice there will be more icons and options than you will actually need with many having dual functions. As the screen changes and you move your cursor[13] (by finger pad or mouse) some options will change. On the next page a numerical reference may help different functions. At the point of repeating the warning, it is important to adopt the discipline of saving material as loss is all too common escalating in emotional responses to varying degrees.

---

[13] Cursor is the arrow that appears on the screen when the mouse pad is moved. It helps to locate the place where you want to travel on the screen.

Saving material

The top bar has a black Apple Logo as shown (left, in the bar diagram). The top bar will disappear when you start to create your slide. Move your cursor up again to bring the information into focus. Software, that is your PowerPoint programme you are working on, will AutoSave, but you can override this and save by clicking the '**save**' icon (5) at any time. The save icon appears to the left of the curly arrow (6) and looks like the old floppy[14] disc. The words, *save this presentation* might appear. The curly arrow allows you to refresh or go back to before the last change. This is very useful if you want to unsave something.

The icon next to the save icon will allow you to create a new file (4). The colour circles to the left of this mean that there are several ways to change the screen. Green (3) means enlarge the screen picture from a smaller size, while the centre (grey) circle (2) allows you to minimise the screen. Closing the file - (1) will prompt you to save before closing the file.

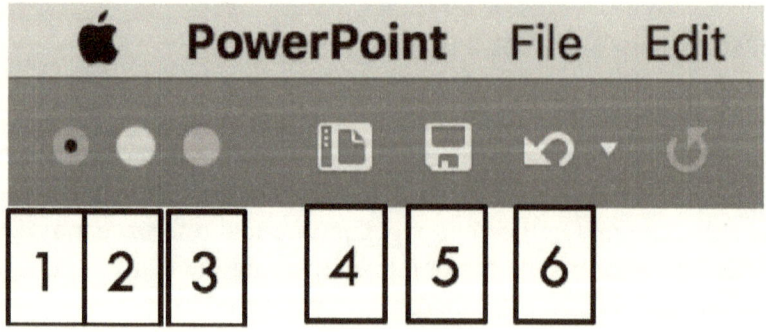

---

[14] Floppy discs were associated with the older drives that saved data and were bendy. The smaller file discs were embedded in harder plastic and a ¼ of the size. As time progressed we moved to USB memory sticks.

Where to save to?

Your file can be saved to different locations. The box shown '**save as**' requires a title i.e My NEW TALK, in the top bar.

The '**where**' to send the file is up to you but if you have a named folder this makes finding the data much easier. Try to label files sensibly with a view to relocating data easily.

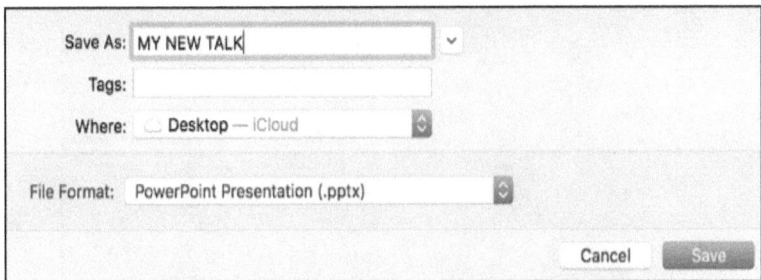

In the slide above, and previously, the location of '**where**' to save was the Desktop. Saving to the desktop is fine but if left there the data size will slow down your computer processing. It is a good idea to save the file to another location on your personal computer as described earlier. Storing files in recognisable folders can make selecting easier. In the next diagram please note that the where above – '**Desktop**' has changed to '**Images folder**' which was a deliberate act to ensure the file is stored somewhere memorable. The folder was created using MY NEW TALK for easier location.

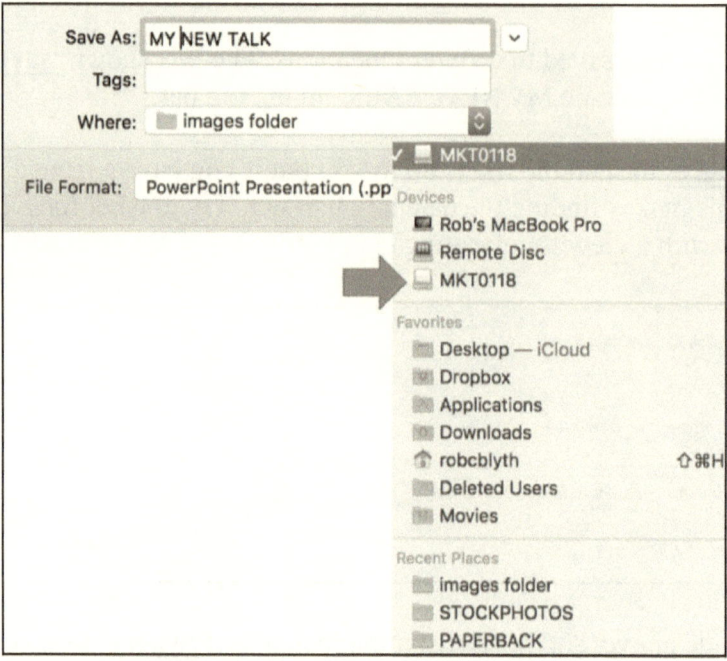

You can save the file to an external device as described earlier. The title called MY NEW TALK can also be saved to a USB flash drive. I have named the flash drive MKT0118 and this will act as an external storage system for my talk. An additional advantage is that I can take it with me to a talk and use it as a back up should my own computer crash, or in the event that I cannot transfer data via the internet to an organiser for my talk. You can save your current slide programme anywhere on the computer using the drop down box created as shown.

Tip: If you lose the location you can use the search facility at the top right hand of the desk top page for the missing file.

Blank Panes

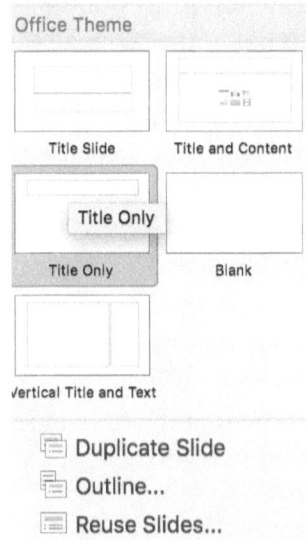

Office Theme

Title Slide

Title and Content

Title Only

Title Only

Blank

Vertical Title and Text

Duplicate Slide

Outline...

Reuse Slides...

A blank pane is the icon or picture represented from eleven options as shown in the table' Office theme' previously under sub-section – options (page 35). The title slide ideally should look attractive as it allows you to set up a title and a subtitle but do remember that you can add your own text box anytime which allows you to place text anywhere on the slide. See over page adding your *free text box*. The illustration opposite is a partial shot of the themes for the 11 blank templates. Notice there is one called 'BLANK' alone and this is often the best one to use to build a slide. Under all of these templates there are three further options and a **'duplicate slide'** option which is very useful and saves copying and pasting[15]. A sub-title provides a little more explanation to support the title but only if required. The top left template indicated '**Title slide**' which you can use if you do not want to use a free text box. See further on for a little more detail under' 'your first title slide' or header slide, (page 44). Pre-formatted slides are less flexible to manipulate but offer faster options for those not wanting a bespoke slide.

---

[15] Pasting implies taking an image or text and moving it and inserting the copied material elsewhere.

It is not important to fine tune your title slide initially. Lay out the first slide as a reference for your draft title. Do not bother with an image at this point, that can be left for later when you feel that an improved title might become apparent as your talk develops. The next line of icons and titles can be seen below. Here we concentrate on the title names. When you click on your text box **'picture format'** appears, adding to the number of options. Each time you move to a different title, the icons will alter the options.

Adding your free text box

The illustration shows a free text box. This can be found either under the **'home'** or **'insert'** icons and so this provides two choices for access.

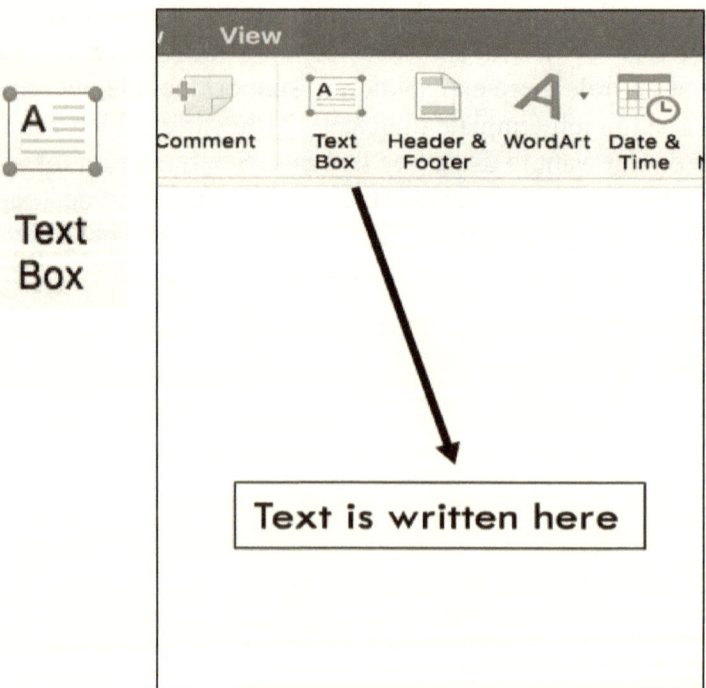

Along the top line with coloured background select **'Insert'**. Find the '**text box**' icon as shown. The two illustrations show that the text box icon has been selected. Move your cursor (the pointer arrow) onto the black space and a small '**A**' on a black background (not shown) appears which you can drag to the position you wish. Click again, the A disappears and a box is seen with four open squares at each corner. By grabbing one corner over the box corner you can stretch out the size to fit and start to type in your text. Just type your text in and arrange the font or size of the words or numbers.

To centre the text (shown on the next page), you will need to go back to '**home**' and this can be found to the left side of insert. Do note that you can access a text box from the '**home**' location or '**insert**' location.

Once you have your text box you can undertake any form of text from titles to lists. You can change the size, colour, design, and font[16], as well as produce a background. Later I will put this altogether to show how titles and text look. It is important not to make text or images fussy as this interfers with the delivery and concentration of any talk. For the moment we need to concentrate on a basic slide deck so we can plan our talk. The illustration on the following page shows four bar lines. This allows sentences and words to centre, move left, right or format evenly as a block. This is the same if you use the Microsoft Word package. The icons shown are self explanatory. Those icons to the right (not shown) provide additional positioning of text.

---

[16] Font means size of the letters for words. 10 is smaller than 12

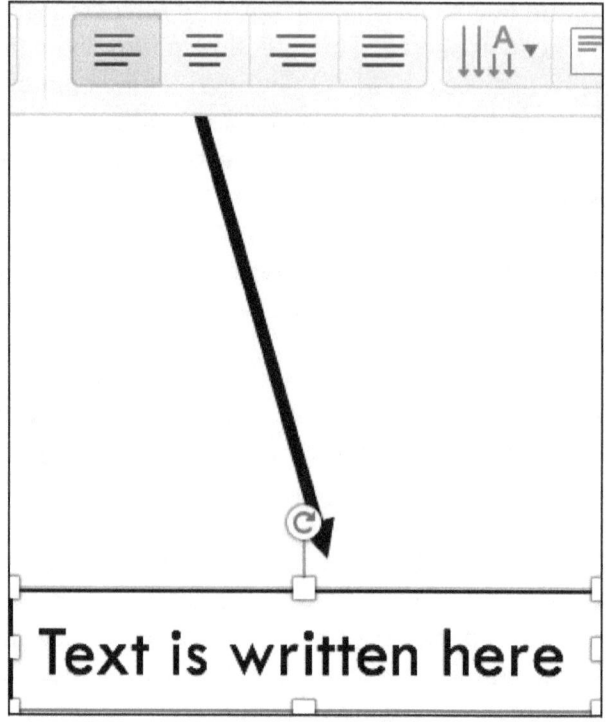

Select 'home' in order to bring the text positioning icons into play. The text written here has been centred.

Your first title slide (Header slide)

I have used '**click to add title and subtitle**' together in the example below to create a working title. This is both punchy and sign posts the subject clearly using four words & numerals. Two examples are described. The fewer words the better. You could make the draft title simpler such as **My trip to Jersey** until you know the angle you want to develop. I am referring to the Channel Islands (UK) and not the state of Jersey, USA. The title could then develop into; **An Island Occupied** if you wanted to look at one aspect of Jersey's history.

I have used a different title in the slide example below. **'Keeping Fit at 50'.** The sub-title contains the author's name (Jane Smith) and her position and company (a fitness club)

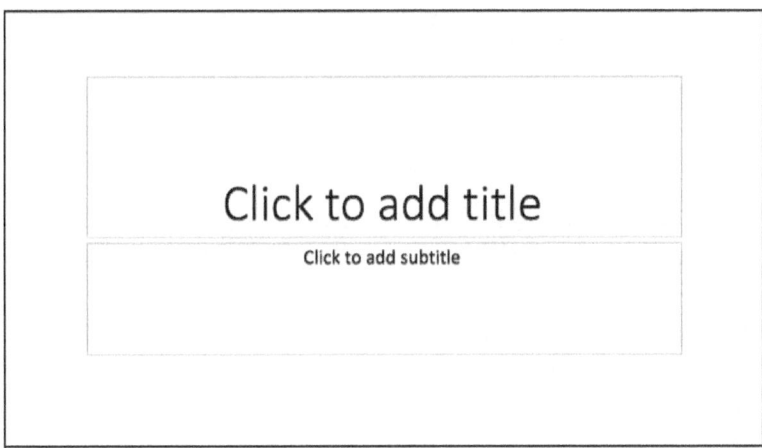

Slide option title + sub-title. Disadvantage. This is best reserved for titles and less user friendly with boxes using bulleted points (see page 57)

(see page 57)

Keeping fit at 50

Jane Smith
Manager, Nobbies Fitness Club

This title slide was created from a text free box allowing the title and sub-title with speaker's position to be promoted in a smaller font. Titles can be created with one of the following options;

Title slide
Title and content
Section header

> **Tip:** If you want to combine titles with picture images stay with a free text box. This will be illustrated later. (Page 61)

Staying with your draft

Now that the idea of using text boxes can be explored, try out a few ideas. As we remain with the theme of planning we need to look at the rest of the content. There are two ways of managing this. Remain with text or go to images as the story board. Of course the other option preferred by some is to write your talk out. Before moving on let's consider the value of writing out the talk.

Writing out your talk

Is this an option?

This part of planning and organising your talk is up to you of course. Writing out your talk helps the order and arrangement of thoughts. Your talk needs a set of philosophical headings as shown in the left hand column of the table on the next page. However, don't use the headings in the table below in your talk but use this idea to develop your structure. There was an old but simplistic adage about speaking:

TELL THEM WHAT YOU ARE GOING TO SAY, SAY WHAT YOU ARE GOING TO SAY AND TELL THEM WHAT YOU HAVE JUST SAID.

Introduction	What am I going to speak about? Main theme. An anecdotal based opening strengthens audience awareness
Middle (content)	Deliver the material you have been working on. Sub-divide the content into a logical order. Maybe divide into three sub themes
End	Your conclusion and highlighting the theme or its subdivisions. The take-away message

Try balancing the 'script'

Here is an example taken from a conference talk that I planned- '*A Look Back …*' as the theme.

I intended to consider the past and contrast it with the present identifying what we still might consider important. The talk was given a time limit of 20 minutes. I wrote the script out and clearly had too much material for 20 minutes. The subject contained confrontation and asked the questions what, how and why. What was the confrontation, how did it impact on each time period and why did it occur? I wrote part of the talk out with these objectives but also built some slides to work out if images could convey material better. You can certainly put up a big question mark on a slide whenever you wish to seek an answer, debate a question or form anything that leads to a query.

A short note in text on your slide might work as a cue within planning your talk but don't make it obvious. Once you have assembled the content you have broken the back of the first part of the talk so can congratulate yourself. You now have manipulated the material into a manageable script. You will need to prune back any unwanted information. But keep any edited material back for later just in case.

The Word processor as with PowerPoint has the advantage of moving or removing redundant material by copying, cutting and pasting. The story board concept works well when trying to arrange your slides in the best order of relevance.

8 - The Story Board

Returning to our theme of planning and the story board, let's look again at the example Jersey, *An Island Invaded*, as the theme. The first thing to do is decide the content and place some text on each slide for outlining your talk. You could do this just as easily on paper, but here we are going to manipulate the slides and convert them to images later on as the talk develops.

There are six slides that provide the spine of the talk. You do not know at this point if you will keep each because you will have to narrow down your key points. The subject is ***island invaded*** and your <u>single</u> story line.

TV Bergerac
Ownership
Invasion and acquisition
Defence and castles
Occupation WW2
Current status

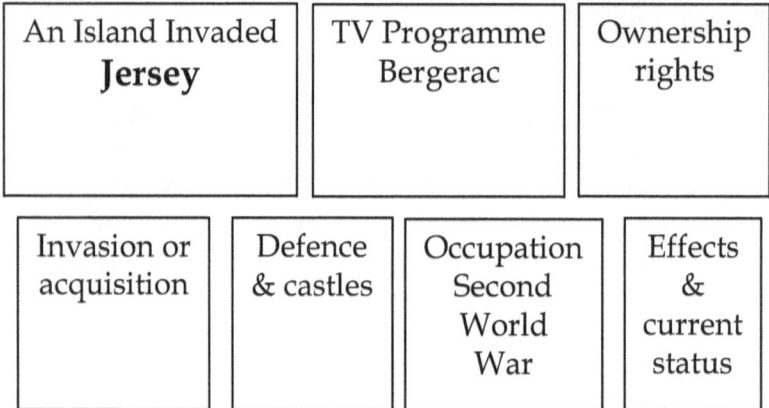

The emphasis lies with invasion and occupation, hence the highlighted line on the framed picture. When planning, use the above as a draft overview rather than the actual slide deck you intend to use. TV Bergerac, shown on the planning board, is not a key point on the story book slide; it is the *hook* upon which we gain the audience's attention. An opportunity to open the talk with a story and draw the audience in. The TV programme, led by John Nettles, was shown between 1981-91.

The Introductory hook

A *hook* is how we bring the audience to full attention and create a parallel subject that bears the hallmarks of a story we call an anecdote based on a fact of interest.

In 2012, the British tabloid, the Daily Mail reported that John Nettles, the lead character in the programme as Jim Bergerac, also playing a fictional police detective on the island of Jersey, made a documentary covering the island during the second world war. As a result, the actor found that he was shunned by islanders when some facts did not act in accordance with their view. *This is the hook*. The story does not contribute to the content per se, but it sets the scene. *The Islanders and their strong sense of identity.*

The slide at the end of the story board contains 'bullets' which provide identity to each sentence. The end slide as with the first slide, called the 'Hook', provides a conclusion and rounds off the talk. If we look for the key elements that must be discussed, then it is occupation during World War 2 (WW2). If we want to make definitive subject points this might be considered around effect and consequence. The background material covering WW2 is extensive and the island has scar lines including a major tourist site around the military hospital built by foreign prisoners. Any peripheral material, such as medieval material would have to be brief or focus on the key times in history when an invasion arose. Too much material will spoil the direction and make the talk less clear as it veers away from the key story line of occupation.

Defence and castles should not be detailed greatly, but ownership would be important as there is a strong Norman-French connection during the first millennium that established an Anglo-French island. Today the island has become a retreat for the wealthy as well as retaining elements of place names in French. The speaker looks for the angle, the twists in a tale and finds anecdotes that resonate to make a good story.

Picture imagery & illustrations?

If we use picture images we should try to establish the provenance of the photo if we are not using our own. Quality plays an important part especially as we need to expand the picture onto a slide. If your picture won't expand without loss of detail, a term called *pixilation*, then use a black background. This is illustrated in the converted 'story board' text to photo images.

Screen grabs

Screen grabs are images that have been essentially lassoed, copied, then pasted onto your slide. The copying feature can be found on most computers. If there is no dedicated button the use of a key board formulae is required. My own Mac Laptops use different sequences to copy an image. Shift-Command-4 would relate to my main PC, but to find how to undertake a screen grab it is best to do a search on-line for your own brand of PC. There are many video films worth clicking on if you are unsure. One useful link includes this one; https://www.take-a screenshot.org/windows.html;

Copyright

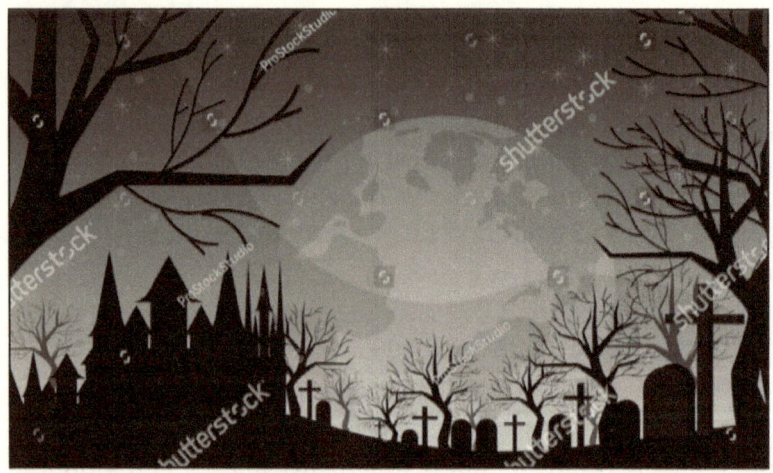

As a guide, any image that has words across the image is copyrighted. Look at the picture of a graveyard[17] with the words *shutterstock* and *ProstockStudio*. This means it requires a license and that implies a payment for the image to be used. There are images which are feely available but do check the status of image copyright before using the image in public.

---

[17] The image shown is actually licensed Shutterstock.com (*on 27.11.19 D. R Tollafield/Busypencilcase Communications Ltd*) produced by ProstockStudio.

—

Story Board slide deck with images

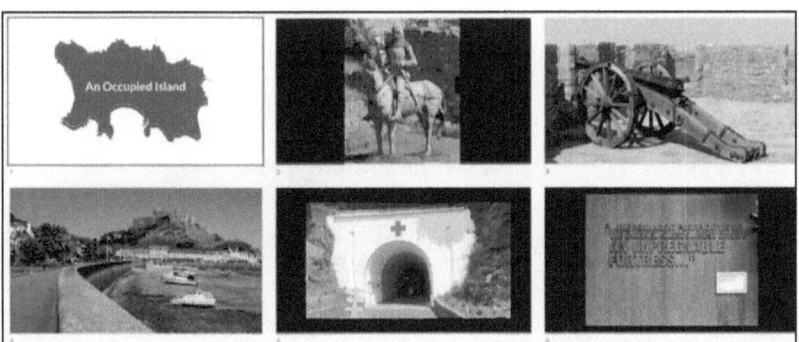

Remaining with the story board theme and planning, the set of slides above replaces the draft text images covering the Jersey Island talk on page 49-50.[18] Six slides have been used again but converted to images. Note the top middle slide has a black background to make up for any loss of detail as I was unable to enlarged the image to cover the whole slide face. The title or header slide now doubles up as a picture and text. This adds interest and sets the scene. The second slide introduces us to a medieval period and defences defined by canon and walled defences of Grosnez castle, Elizabeth castle and Mont Orgueil castle. The underground hospital is important and conveys the horrors of Nazi occupation. The last slide, a picture of an embossed dedication plate would be suited to closing the talk.

Because the story board is part of planning, more slides would be anticipated for a 40-minute talk. The value derived from images is that they work well with narrative and the speaker can discuss a range of different plots and themes as long as the image fits the theme being discussed.

---

[18] Toursist pictures taken from internet free stock. Map of Jersey licensed as L.N. Vector Pattern/Shutterstock.com

Avoiding complex text

While discussing the story board it is likely that you will retain a number of slides created as the story board for the final talk. In order to minimise duplication of effort it is important to consider some of the rules early on rather than introduce them at the end.

There are two fundamental reasons not to write large amounts of text on a slide. The first reason is that your audience will read the material and not listen to your words of wisdom. The text will also no doubt diminish in size so as not to be seen clearly if sentences are used. The second reason relates to the quality of your talk. Although I have suggested text offers an aid memoire, it is better to work off a supplementary card during the presentation to keep the delivery in order. Images will also keep you organised so you relate any memorised text to the slide. The flow of delivery (spoken word) will remain interrupted if rather than reading the text, the audience focuses on as few written words as possible while trying to listen.

RULE
Use the least text required.
Substitute images relating to your narrative.
Only use text to deliver the key point you wish to make.
Never write text out in full.
Do not use a slide (text or otherwise image) to say what you are about to say.
Try to use text after speaking to reinforce your point so your audience listens before reading.

Text writing should be left to the cue note section below the slide. You can write effusively here as no-one will see this, unless you publish your PowerPoint. It is common in conferences to be asked to allow the organisers to use your lecture slides. BE CAREFUL when sharing slides.

TIP: You may have written rough notes at the bottom of a slide but the language can be misinterpreted when read out of context. Remove any text under the slide, even though it is hidden, OR vet it carefully.

DO NOT give permission to use your slides if they are not yours, or where material is licensed or original and you want to use the material elsewhere. Unless you are paid for your material or services which includes the slide material, this is yours. Licensed material may include purchased images from IT companies. You have the license; anyone who copies this and uses it does not.

Bergman's Milestones

Bergman points out that when we travel, *I use the example Manchester to Liverpool (UK)*, we use signs that inform us of distance. The information assumes the digital '35'. We would not read a sign that says,

THE DISTANCE FROM MANCHESTER TO LIVERPOOL IS
THIRTY-FIVE MILES

The fact that the data values are miles in the UK or USA does not matter as this is a given. Thirty-five ('35 miles') would be easier to read rapidly and understood than words, i.e **Manchester to Liverpool 35 miles**. Bergman recommends having a maximum of 4 words on the slide for the purpose of text as a milestone. Anymore and the reader will not grab the message quickly. When fewer words are used the size of the text can be made larger and easier to see.

I have attended so many talks where my mind wanders. Perhaps I am tired and drift away thinking of another problem, but the fault is not always mine. Engagement with the audience is essential and the ingredients of any talk come down to the nuts and bolts. If the structure and delivery is carefully designed it is possible to maintain the audience's engagement. If the audience has no interest to start with and the place of the meeting is a convenient place to hide from the family or rain, well then no-one can predict the effect of an unfamiliar topic. Nonetheless, I have listened to many radio programmes that were entitled dull as dust but the content was engaging.

> **RULE:** Use an image instead of text to associate your narrative. Make sure the image relates to the narrative but does not copy or replicate the narrative

---

EXAMPLE OF WORKING NARRATIVE WITH IMAGE

POOR
Image - red bus.
Narrative - most buses are red.

BETTER
Image - red bus with advertisement.
Narrative - double decker buses have caught on throughout most of the world as the advertising industry and tourist trade recognises the intrinsic value of their size and capacity. The mobility of the bus and travelling advert has advantages over a stationary advert because of the number of people that the advert can reach. There is no mention of the colour red.

The image could show size, and maybe an advert. The audience will not have thought of this, but would know this if they considered the advantages of the bus advert.

The link with tourism is that more seats equals more income, not convenience for the tourist. Buses are also able to enjoy larger adverts at the back as well as the sides. The point I am making is that while you are saying something similar it is not the same. An image should reinforce the narrative.

An example of complex text

While there is an appetite amongst may speakers to use complex text, it is important not to dominate a slide. Consider the milestone approach recommended by Bergman and avoid creating large numbers of lists. An alternative way to use a list like approach is to slide one line of text in, talk to the heading and then introduce a second. This is called animation as distinct from transitioning. In this way the audience can read and listen as the milestone approach starts to work visually. There is a tendency to reproduce large sections of text. Such acts probably derive from false assumptions and trying to comfort oneself that you have covered all the material on the slide. Don't!

You might feel that Abraham Lincoln's Gettysburg address would be important to reproduce but it is important to compose text with limited information even when planning. This avoids the temptation to read the text, but when using the represented as bullet points. Here is an example. Although Lincoln's speech was short, there are 271 words in the text. The speech stood for freedom and honour against the backdrop of hard battle. Equally you could represent the text with bulleted points as below:

- All men are created equal
- (They) gave their lives
- Birth of Freedom

'Four score and seven years ago our fathers brought forth on this continent, a new nation, conceived in Liberty, and dedicated to the proposition that all men are created equal. Now we are engaged in a great civil war, testing whether that nation, or any nation so conceived and so dedicated, can long endure. We are met on a great battle-field of that war. We have come to dedicate a portion of that field, as a final resting place for those who here gave their lives that that nation might live. It is altogether fitting and proper that we should do this. But, in a larger sense, we can not dedicate -- we can not consecrate -- we can not hallow -- this ground. The brave men, living and dead, who struggled here, have consecrated it, far above our poor power to add or detract. The world will little note, nor long remember what we say here, but it can never forget what they did here. It is for us the living, rather, to be dedicated here to the unfinished work which they who fought here have thus far so nobly advanced. It is rather for us to be here dedicated to the great task remaining before us -- that from these honored dead we take increased devotion to that cause for which they gave the last full measure of devotion -- that we here highly resolve that these dead shall not have died in vain -that this nation, under God, shall have a new birth of freedom -- and that government of the people, by the people, for the people, shall not perish from the earth.'

Abraham Lincoln. November 19, 1863

A slide with bullets could be animated for each line separately to cover the historical implication. *Animations and transitions* will be dealt with later in chapter 15 and offer a way of limiting the distraction for the audience by allowing only the words that you want to appear visible while talking. There is an additional method of presenting text again using Lincoln's speech. In this case scenario only the key words show in bold while the remaining text is lighter using a grey colour. The slide shows the magnitude of words but highlights the key themes that Lincoln was driving at.

Four score and seven years ago our fathers brought forth on this continent, a new nation, conceived in Liberty, and dedicated to the proposition that **all men are created equal**. Now we are engaged in a great civil war, testing whether that nation, or any nation so conceived and so dedicated, can long endure. We are met on a great battle-field of that war. We have come to dedicate a portion of that field, as a final resting place for those who here **gave their lives** that that nation might live. It is altogether fitting and proper that we should do this.

But, in a larger sense, we can not dedicate -- we can not consecrate -- we can not hallow -- this ground. The **brave men, living and dead,** who struggled here, have consecrated it, far above our poor power to add or detract. The world will little note, nor long remember what we say here, but it can never forget what they did here. It is for us the living, rather, to be dedicated here to the unfinished work which they who fought here have thus far so nobly advanced. It is rather for us to be here dedicated to the great task remaining before us -- that from these honored dead we take increased devotion to that cause for which they gave the last full measure of devotion -- that we here highly resolve that these dead shall not have died in vain -- that this nation, under God, shall have a new **birth of freedom -- and that government of the people, by the people, for the people, shall not perish from the earth.**

Speech, Abraham Lincoln, November 19, 1863.

9 - Bullet Points

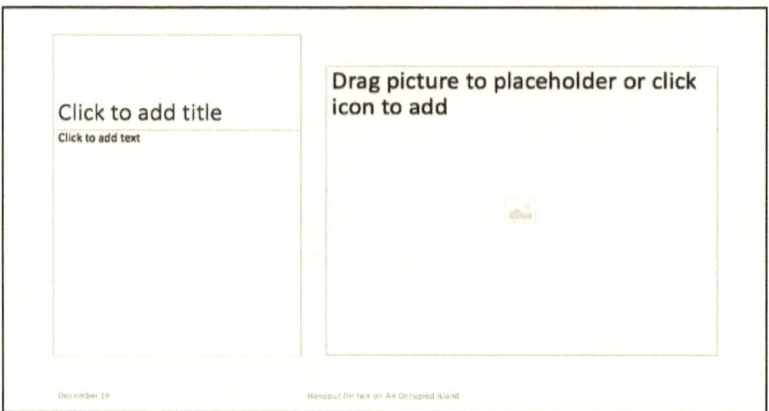

Template for title, sub-title and a picture

In written works bullet points allow words to have order and emphasis. This is not the same visually. However, any summary may use *bullet points* to produce recapitulation which may also be repeated during the course of the talk. Those little shapes to the left of the lines come as black dots, dashes, diamonds and so on. Their purpose is to attract attention and appear as a great way to deliver lectures. But, when all is said and done they are created by the speaker rather than for the audience. The use of bullets in teaching is valuable when the class can make notes, if required, and the points should be dropped down in a sequence to marry with the narrative or your spoken word. It should be noted that a free text box is the best way to ensure bullet points can be utilised. Some preformed title blank templates will not allow bullets. Look at the blank template for a **'picture** *created* **with caption'** from the options list above. This uses mixed images of text+title+illustration as a handout page. Note the borders are created so that you can populate each separately. The template sets the font initially although this can still be altered.

Bullets are used in the lower left hand box where **'<u>click to add text</u>'** is indicated. Chris Davidson calls the use of bullets *'the highest ranking crime of audience abuse,'* the bullet point conflicts with the audiences' senses and suggests the brain cannot multi-task. Anything that causes your audience to switch off means you lose them. While the example associated with the Lincoln speech does not look too heavy, once altered many speakers have a tendency to create long lists. Look at the list below as an example of a reasonable

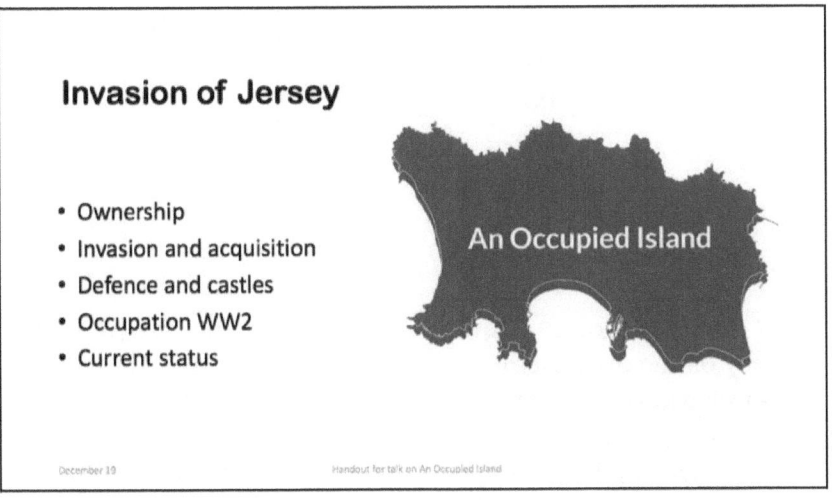

Map Jersey/L.N.VectorPattern

presentation.

In the next slide (over the page) there are no bullets but a list. To create impact it would be better to show the slide with **'<u>Land</u>'** alone, then *forestry*, and drop down each label thereafter while speaking. In this manner the audience can focus on the necessary text. So often speakers dump text, speak and move on. The listener is still scribbling as the next slide comes up. Use one point per slide.

Land

  forestry
  rivers / lakes
  hills / mountains
  villages/towns/cities

Coastline

  estuaries
  rivers
  tides
  sea

Speakers often say, you can download my lecture from my website, or they rely on the organiser to send the PowerPoint. While useful our lives move at such a pace that messages can be lost and time fails to allow well intentioned follow up. The slide covering a list of geographic areas might be used at the end to compile the overall picture. I am not a critic of the bullet list but I strongly argue for easy to read slides and the way they are delivered in a talk no matter what speaking style. Few can follow complex slides and listen without prior knowledge.

> **TIP:** Keep bullets the same size and design throughout the slide deck. Use bullet points and lists **after** speaking from a blocker slide (page 68).
> The speaker is advised to learn the order of delivery and not rely on the list.
> Use cues in the form of hand size cards to aid delivery.

'YOUR VISUAL AIDS SHOULD SUPPLEMENT YOUR STORY;
NOT THE OTHER WAY AROUND.' ERIC BERGMAN

An overpopulated slide, whether using text, images or both form a cardinal sin. Slide design is not just for artistic creation.

ANOTHER RULE: ONE SLIDE = ONE IDEA

There are a great many ways to use PowerPoint and all its facilities but concentrating on a basic format makes sense. Style, colour, background form the principle components. In time you can experiment and add to the basics with experience. Mac and Microsoft PCs both use the PowerPoint system although the packages have to be bought individually. Every time an upgrade comes out the navigation changes and so it is not feasible to say all PowerPoint packages are the same. Do check the screen set up on your slide programme because at conferences you will be requested to use a specific format.

Select 'design' and then follow the bar to the right[19] and locate the icon below; **<u>'Slide Size'</u>**. See the illustrated screen grab over the page.

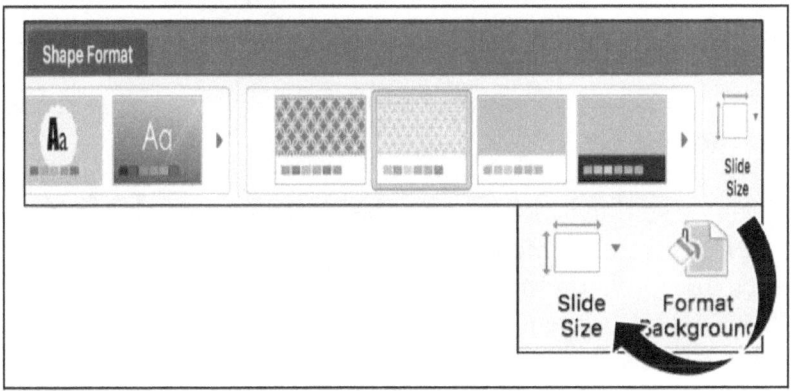

---

[19] The illustrated screen grab has been made to show the important icons and is not a true representation of the view you will actually see.

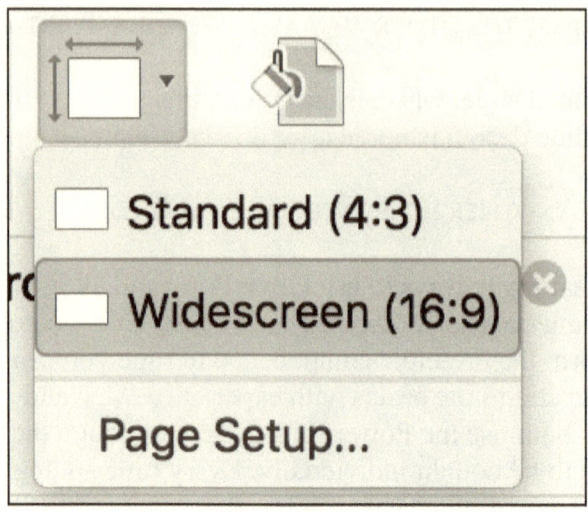

The remaining icons on the bar (page 61) are colour options. The size of the slide is either in a square or rectangle format. This can be changed at any time but the **Page Setup** icon will provide Standard (4:3), Widescreen (16:9) or Widescreen (16:10). The latter value is on an older PowerPoint package while the newer ones may have the first two options of size. Of course this is a generalisation and PowerPoint will be updated constantly over time. But, doubtless we keep our old programmes for longer periods than the designers would like.

Does size matter?

If your laptop setting is not right for the screen you may lose the edges of the picture. Conference organisers will know the format and may even ask for that format based on the above ratios. Elsewhere you may need to change it depending on the screen you are projecting against.

WordArt

As we are still talking text (words) I will bring in WordArt. We will need to consider the icons first so we select **'insert'** and the following icon bar will appear. Some of the icons to the right have been left out purely as they are surplus to need at this point. The bar is shown below and then enlarged to identify the key icons used. WordArt appears at the far right side of this illustration (**12**).

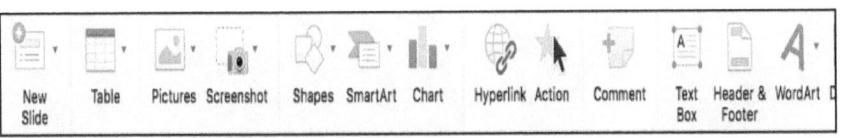

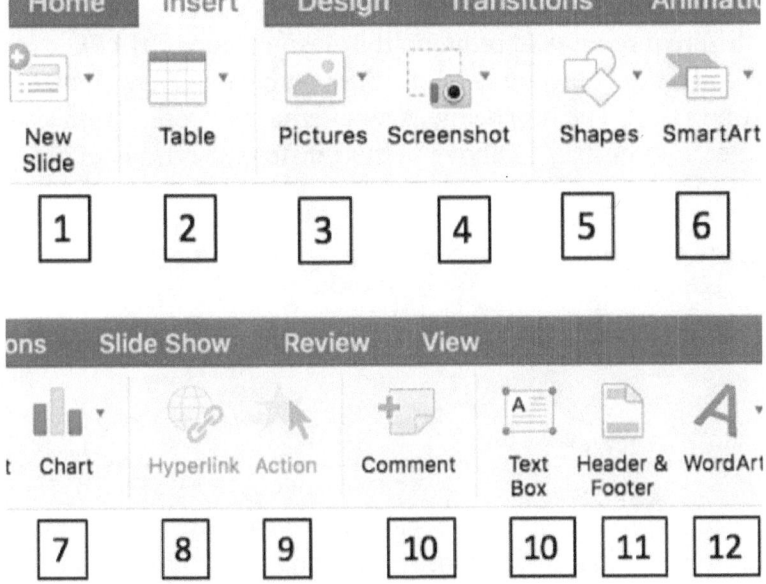

During planning, and perhaps later when the slide deck is finalised we will also use **Table (2)**, **Pictures (3)**, **Shapes (5)**, **SmartArt (6)**, **Charts (7)**, **Text box (10)**.

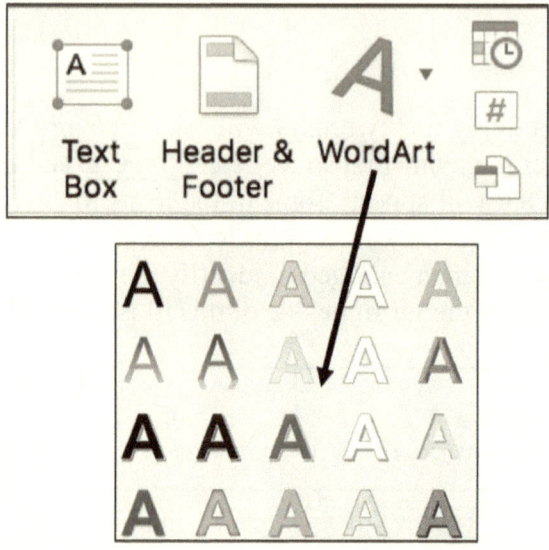

WordArt (12) used to be separately named and you may have to select a different process to bring up this design called SHAPE FORMAT. To select this on version 15.8 you have to have created your text box first. The box below is an alternative presentation while the picture of the A's above in their different styles is in the expanded box.

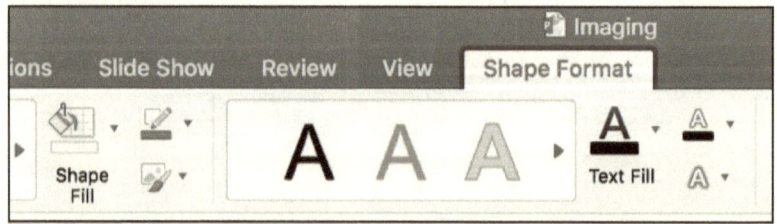

Try not to mix styles, keep to one that does the job. Be consistent. The style of words has colour (not shown) and an outline to make it stand out.

This is WordArt

Generally, when we present a slide the room should not be in darkness or subdued to enhance the slides. At the start of chapter 2, Jabber, Jabber, the old style projector often needed the curtains closed or lights dimmed. This can be a disaster as it can send audiences to sleep. So when I talk about darkness on a slide we need to be alive to the fact we should not dive the room into a black morass.

A word from Actor Mark Strong[20]

Mark Strong's clear booming voice could be heard at the start of the scheduled film. The value of darkness is understated as it allows the audience more concentration because there is no distraction. Making the start count is important.

'Hello,
Makes you notice doesn't it?
A little bit of darkness.
Refines the senses. Focuses the mind.
It's time to enjoy the big screen experience with NO distractions, sudden ring tones, NO glaring screens, NO talking.
So sit back and relax.
Switch off your phone and switch off from the outside world'

---

[20] Strong (Vue Cinemas, 2019) was asked to narrate an introduction for different film classifications. This has been updated for 2020 with images. The passage can be found on YouTube.

10 - The Blocker slide

Of all the slides that you might create, the blocker slide is actually the most valuable. First it is important to say what it is. **Slide 21** of course is the slide in question. Two of the slides also show a black background, with **slide 22** with white writing, but the main background is white;

'LIKE ANY ADDICTION POWERPOINT IS DIFFICULT TO STOP.' ERIC BERGMAN.

Slide 24 is an image slide depicting a boat. This slide is in fact an anecdote and inside the boat a lecture facility appears in the story about an itinerant speaker who broke some cardinal rules.
Slide 23 is a text slide or text image which states 'READING'. In the case of slide 22 & 23, the point about the two slides is to show that reading a slide makes poor use of your skills. The delivery of the same words would be better on a black blocker slide. Using the slide 22 later might be of better value as recapitulation. The blocker will prevent any image being visible to the audience and as a result will divert their attention to you the speaker. Your words will carry optimum impact and any distraction will be minimised. Your aim is to ensure at this point your message gains greatest recognition and is recalled. During planning allow your deck of slides to be punctuated with a break, i.e a blocker slide. You know that you need to insert spoken words in here and we will for the moment call these free text slides. This means you should be able to speak without any aids at this point removing any distraction from the audience. There is one big problem with a blocker slide and that is ensuring that you know

a) what the next slide will show
b) that you do not accidently hit that slide using your control button.

If you do accidently knock on the next slide, try to reverse as quickly as you can and say nothing but carry on. <u>Do not</u> draw attention to your minor mistake.

Tip: avoid apologising unless absolutely necessary.
Other examples include;
- 'Sorry this picture is not clear!'
- 'I forgot to put the video clip in!'
- 'We'll come to this shortly!' *This is fine once but not if it provides a repetitive feature when talking*
- 'The explanation is too difficult, or I've not got enough time allotted!'
- I'm nearly finished, do you mind if we use part of your coffee break! *One of the worst crimes is stealing time from your audience.*

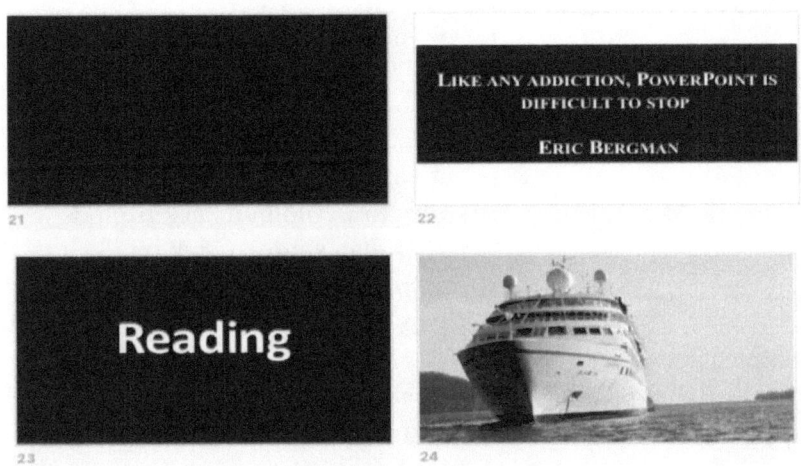

These excuses have all been trotted out before and the point being made is that if you had planned and prepared, such events should not happen. Take care of the minor errors as well as the obvious ones that should not occur. Above all do not blame others.

How to make a blocker slide?

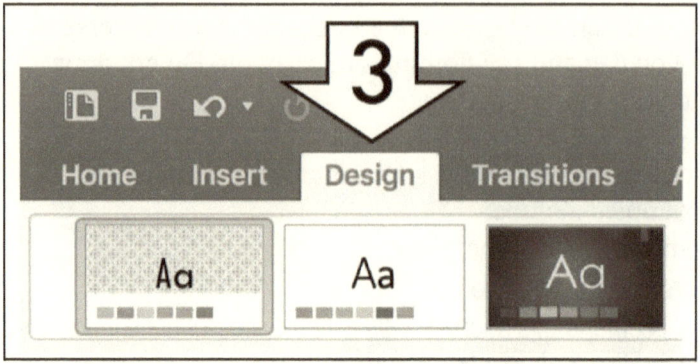

There are two ways to make a black background based slide.
Use the design title icon (3) or click on the slide itself (right mouse click) and select **format background** as shown.

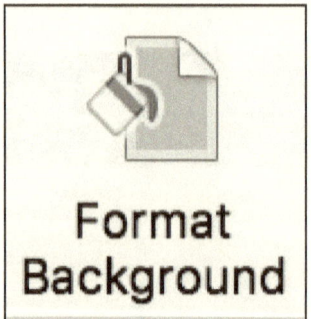

The **Design slide** is faster than using the mouse with **format background** but the choice lies with you and what works for you. The design slide if activated as a label will convert all slides to a coloured background rather than singly. Click on (3) *design* and you will see a selection of panes arise above the slide or use the icon above showing a tipping paint pot. If you use **format background** the illustration shown at the bottom of the next page shows the dropdown menu with a number of options. The design slide using black **Aa** is instant colour application.

Find the black slide, click on the **Aa icon** and the white blank will change colour to black. When using the format background option further options open to the right. Part of your slide will disappear when the column appears. The drop down box provides solid fill option (bullet marked) but the colour bar must be changed to black (or any other choice) to effect this alteration.

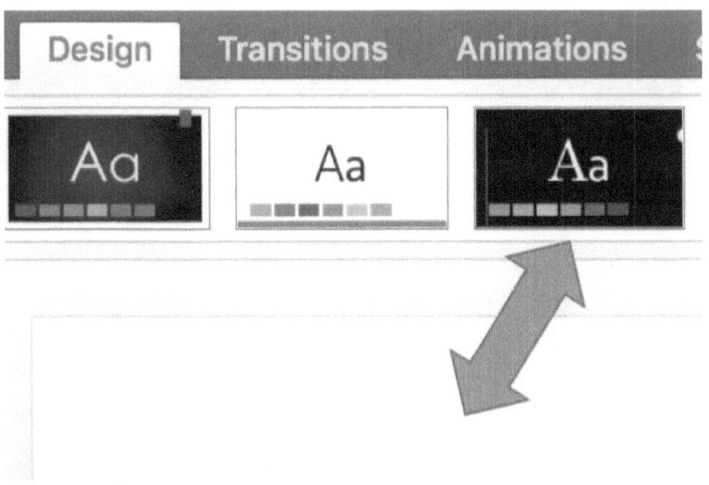

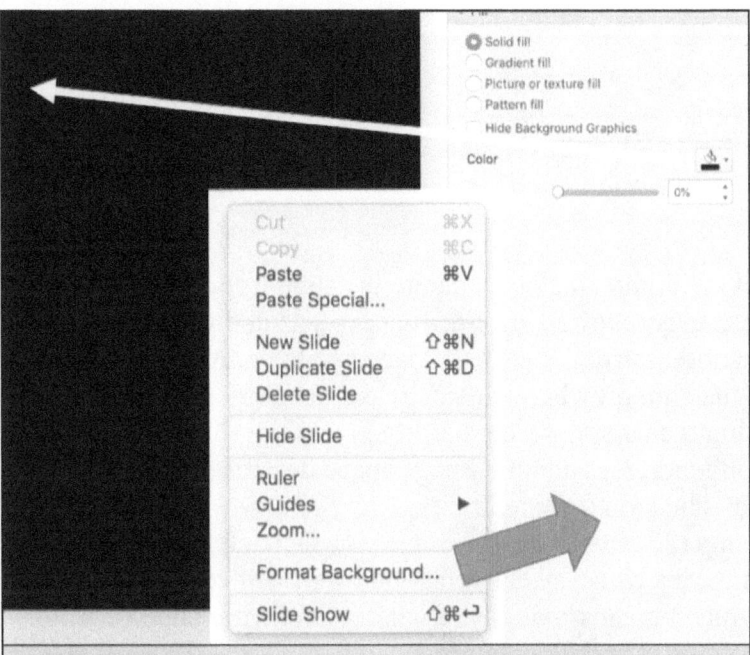

While I have talked about the blocker or black slide, it is possible to use other colours. White is often selected as a background. It should be pointed out why black is best. It does not reflect as much as creates better attention. A white slide is bright and glares. If we consider Mark Strong's words; 'no glaring screens' now makes sense.

Notes for slides

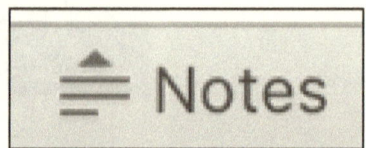

Earlier we considered planning your slides as a story board as well as writing out the talk as options. One of the facilities that PowerPoint offers is the use of the **'add notes'** option. This provides an additional method of creating cues during your practice runs.

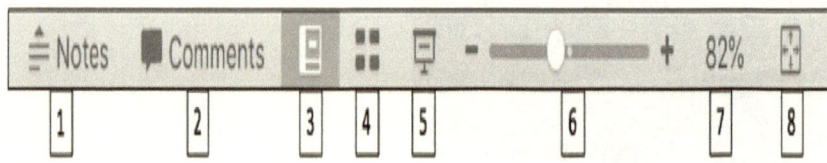

Notes (1) will immediately separate the slide from an area below to allow you to type text. The slide reduces size and you can manually increase or diminish the writing space available. Alternatively, you can use the slim grey bar that sits below the slide and lifting up the slide using the cursor. As the bar lifts, two things happen. The space for writing increases and the image space decreases (see illustration opposite– click to add notes).

Comments (2) can be ignored but if you share slide programmes you can have a two-way conversation by way of editing slides and making recommendations if you wish to send your slide deck to someone else as in collaboration.

Altering the screen (3) will open up a side bar showing all the slides currently designed.

Four squares (4) shows the slides in horizontal order. Both 3 and 4 will allow you to move slides around into a different position. This provides a fast method of editing order.

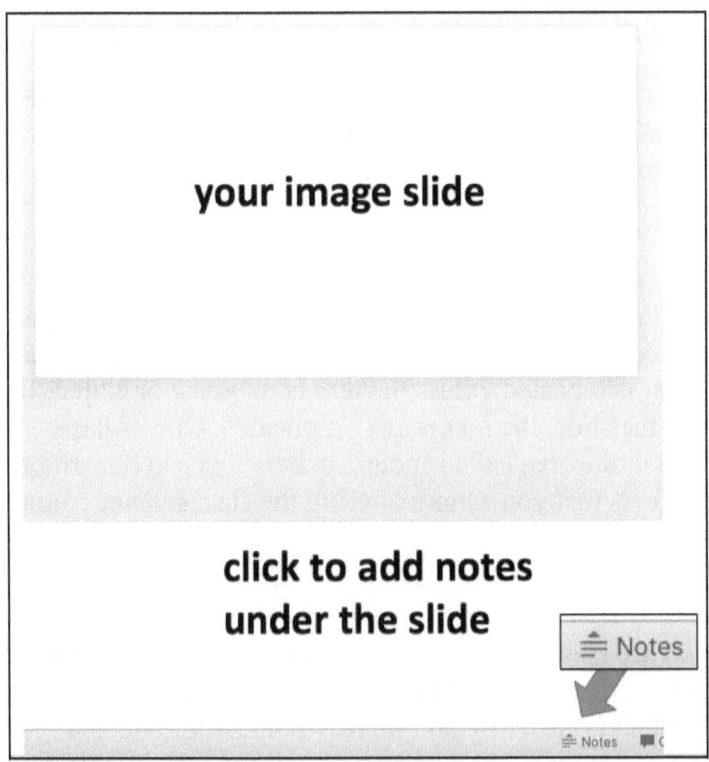

The image of the slide above shows the screen has split into two elements. A blank slide format **'your image slide'** and a **'click to add notes'**. The operations bar highlighting **'notes'** can be seen below with a grey background.

PowerPoint viewer (5) the slide view is the same view that your audience will see, i.e only the image shown is of the slide itself without any surrounding information
The image size to screen (6) the slide bar runs from negative to positive values and will allow you to increase or decrease each slide viewed as in 3 & 4 to make viewing and editing easier. The percentage gain or loss is shown in numerical form with a % sign (7). By clicking on the four arrows in box icon (8) the screen defaults back to 100%.

<u>Recording</u> You can type as normal or dictate using the **fn key** to record (Macs). There is usually a slight lag with the dictation facility before the words appear.

<u>Duplication</u>
Additionally, you can take any section from your written script or layout in Word, then copy and paste this into the space so you only write it out once. The text now resides with that slide. If the slide is copied, the text is repeated unless the text is removed or edited. If you duplicate the slide, the text is also duplicated. One of the downsides about the area called 'notes', where text can be written below the slide, is that you cannot altering the size, style or colour.

Overall aim

Although you are concentrating on designing a talk, your aim is to hone all the narrative down to bite size chunks. By drilling down words the content is easier to handle. Key points (not bulleted points) act as a shopping list to help you memorise the important elements required for your talk. You can also write the key points on the back of hand held cue cards. If your projector goes down or a bulb pops, the cue card provides a replacement and a welcome rescue aid.

Part 3
The Last Stages

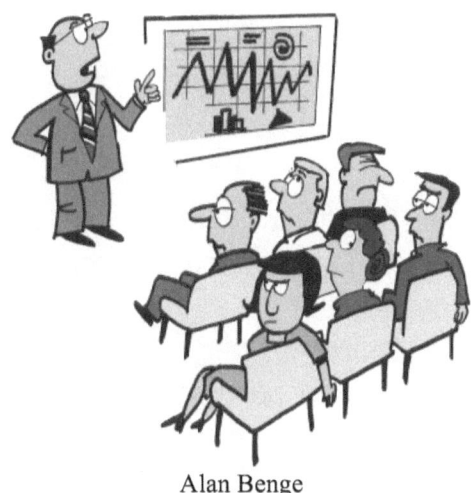

Alan Benge

Learning about all the elements of any system may seem laborious and certainly there is no substitute than practice. Make mistakes by all means as that is how we learn. Never feel afraid to experiment, but perhaps do not overcomplicate your slide deck as you will have plenty to do just concentrating on talking to the audience. In part 3 it is useful to draw together the building blocks created so far. As your new blocks are created your structure will strengthen. Once you have planned your story board you need to broaden your horizons and start putting all the bricks in place to create a firm foundation.

The fable of the three little pigs withstanding the big bad wolf comes to mind with their robust brick built house. Anything less robust will fall down. Unlike fables we can look to the morale behind stories and this one is true.

'Here are my slides, can you cover my talk?'

When a speaker could not attend a conference he loaned his lecture to another colleague to talk on the same subject. Both of equal ability and good speakers. This is the summary of what happened to the second stand-in speaker:

The Story
He had no time to plan.
Was unfamiliar with the slide content and sequence.
His narrative floundered as he stopped to consider in real time what the slide meant.
The narrative failed to flow.
Being unaware of the rule of points he failed to highlight the aims of the talk.
Because of different thoughts and interpretations, the material did not synchronise with the slides.

IF YOU ARE TO COVER SOMEONE ELSE'S PRESENTATION YOU STILL HAVE TO PREPARE AND DESIGN YOUR TALK.

We need to assemble the loose nuts and bolts into a formal structure. The principles of talking to small informal or large meetings remain the same. The effort taken is proportional to the success of the talk. Success therefore comes from preparation.

By creating a natural appearance of ease with your delivery represents the second benefit from steady preparation. With practise the recovery of the words you wish to use during your talk become more accessible and mistakes, fluffs or stumbles are ironed out and less likely to arise.

11 - Making Imagery Work

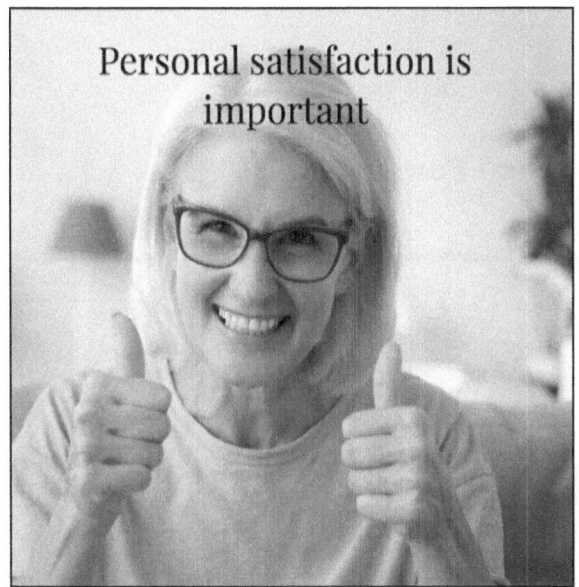

Personal satisfaction is important

Fizkes/Shutterstock.com

'THE MOST IMPORTANT THING TO REMEMBER IS THAT THE SLIDES ARE NOT THE CONTENT SO NEVER READ FROM THEM. THEY SHOULD BE SUPPORT FOR THE TALK, OR FOR THE VISUAL EFFECT.' - JOANNA PENN

As a speaker I want to look at any facility that can help me. My memory may not be as good as it was once although as we age we recall earlier history better than recent events. So the slide can act as a cue.

Joanna Penn points out you should be able to speak without slides if the technology goes wrong. So when preparing your talk consider what will happen if your images fail. How will you cope? The tip of making a print-out of your slides, which we will call the **slide deck**, is sensible.

Cue cards and PowerPoint

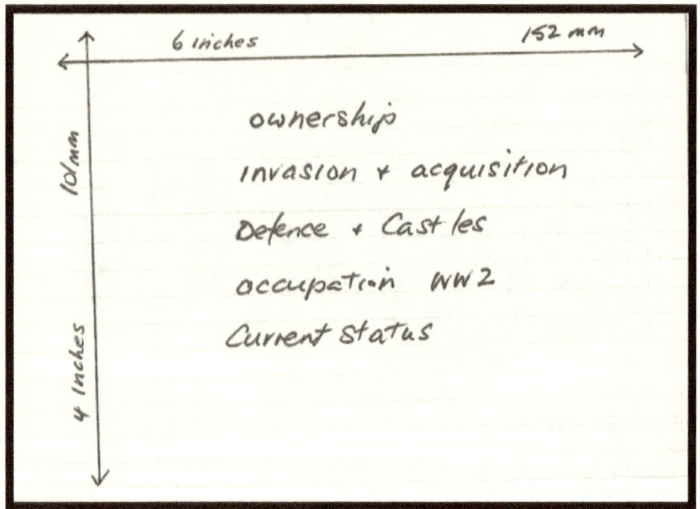

Cue cards act as memory aids; the one above measure 6x4 in or 152x101mm. The actor Antony Hancock became dependent on cue cards toward the end of his acting career and many talented people use cues to help order their words. There is nothing wrong with this but PowerPoint can help produce a physical card saving you some effort.

You can also print out a sheet of slides for yourself as much as you can create a handout for your audience.

Summary: text & images

Too many images
Create a further slide page so the image is not crowded.
Use animations and transitions to break up the overcrowding effect.

Over-populated text
This forms the largest of all the cardinal sins and there are no apologies for repeating the message.
The reason speakers put too much writing on a slide is that they want to read the slide as it contains information for their talk.
Too many proceed to read from the slide.
DO speak using the cue card as a prompt.
Lengthy text leaves the audience distracted; switched off to listening.
Bullet points are the lesser evil and if transitioned are more acceptable as described.
Where notes are not available, the speaker should pause, to allow notes to be taken. Consider the audience within planning.

Graphs
Represent data. You can actually use a table to represent data but complex tables are harder to read than simple pie and bar charts which excel at showing growth trends visually.
In academic circles these facilities are helpful but so often even clever researchers put up busy graphs which provide too much overlap information. ONE SLIDE PER IDEA
The idea behind showing data is to show how it contributes to change, emphasising narrative.
Show a graph rather than a table.
Highlight the areas of most interest, or add colour to the cells.
Diminish data-text if not needed so it pales in colour & contrast.
Grey colours leave the black to stand out.
The other method of presenting data is to only use valid figures of most value.
Data needs to be explained and reasons given for representing data on the slide.

Printing off the slide deck

You can have up to 9 slides per page. Printing is provided by a drop down box that provides options when **'printer'** is selected. Here are the steps:

Select **FILE**

From the drop down box select **PRINT**

Within the print box there will be a heading: **PRINT WHAT**.
Select this and it will tell you to select handouts for example (2 – 9 slides per page)

Once selected, an image shows what will be printed.

Cue card with brief information to jog one's memory and keep order. Of course you need to know the content!

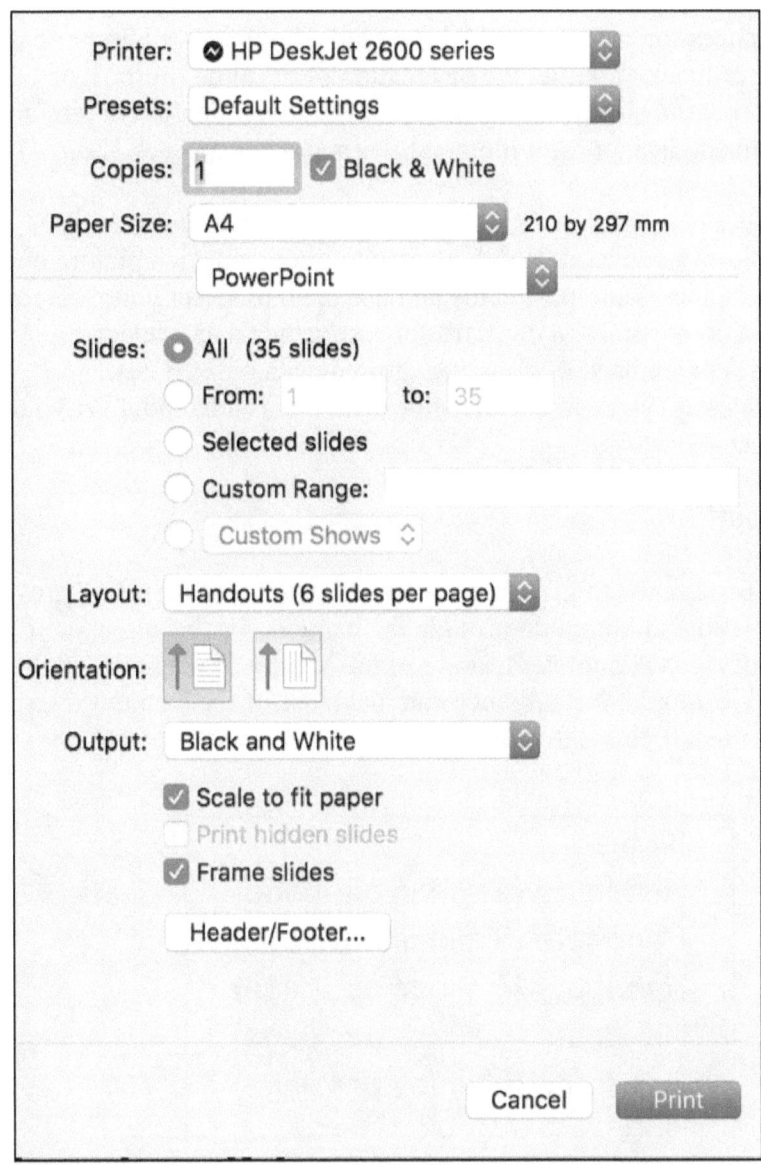

The PowerPoint slide deck can be printed off to form cue card. Insert your preferences in the boxes

Preferences for running off slides include number of slides per page, colour or black & white, the orientation of the slide (portrait or landscape) not shown in this image but can be found to the left, and you can add headers and footers, titles and dates on each slide.

Six slides per A4 is about right where the image is sufficiently readable as a cue card. You have the option to cut each picture out and paste them onto post cards and use them to select your preferred order. You now have a cue card for emergency and a selector facility. On the back of your cue card you can make notes. Alternatively, you can use the slide print out as a handout for your audience.

Handout[21]

Don't be tempted to give this out before your talk as it might provide a distraction, although do provide the handout for the audience if you wish them to take notes. Because of the brevity of the slides in the 'Island' example, the audience can make use of the handout if issued before the talk to make notes.

```
Slides
Handouts (2 slides per page)
Handouts (3 slides per page)
Handouts (4 slides per page)
Handouts (6 slides per page)
Handouts (9 slides per page)
Notes
✓ Outline
```

---

[21] Handouts: These should supplement notes related to the talk and can contain references for further reading. Avoid too much detail and highlight key themes only.

If you want the audience to take notes provide a handout before the talk. If the handout is intended to be detailed, then leave it to the end of the talk.

If you select 'Outline' from the drop down menu (see the printed sheet below) you can produce a different handout or aid as a cue sheet listing all the text but the images

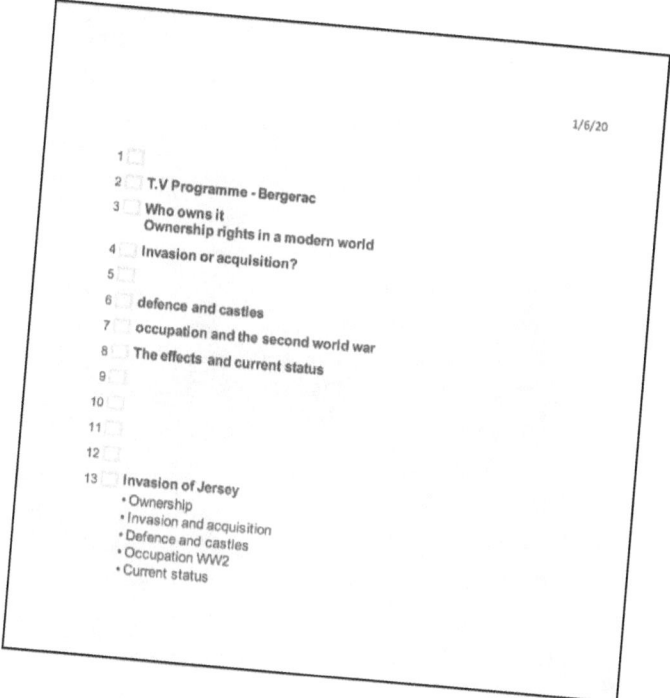

1,5,7,9-12 for the 13 listed slides are missing because pictorial images are not captured.

12 - Connecting with your audience

Websites and internet

If you are a serious speaker and feel you want to keep in touch with your audience, or indeed offer the audience something for attending, a handout or leaflet is something that can be appreciated. If you are pitching to sell, then this may become more important.

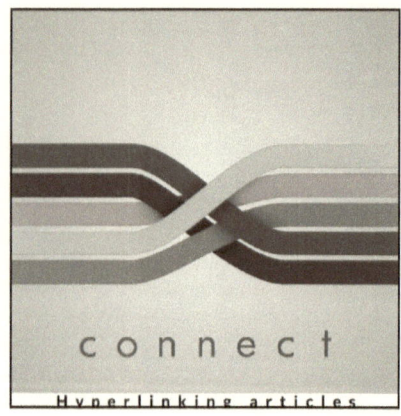

'ClickHere'

Support your audience

Anticipate that your audience may want to find the information and undertake their own research. You can provide a list of sources. As we exist in a world of fast communication the value behind e-handouts served by the internet may be better. Remember that many e-mail address providers set a limit on the number of addresses that can be used even if you are using them under the blind carbon copy (BCC) option.

A Mailer system is recommended and some of these provide a free service up to a certain number of users. Text can be hyperlinked to sources that connect directly to the internet. Audiences today are less patient than those even from the 20th century.

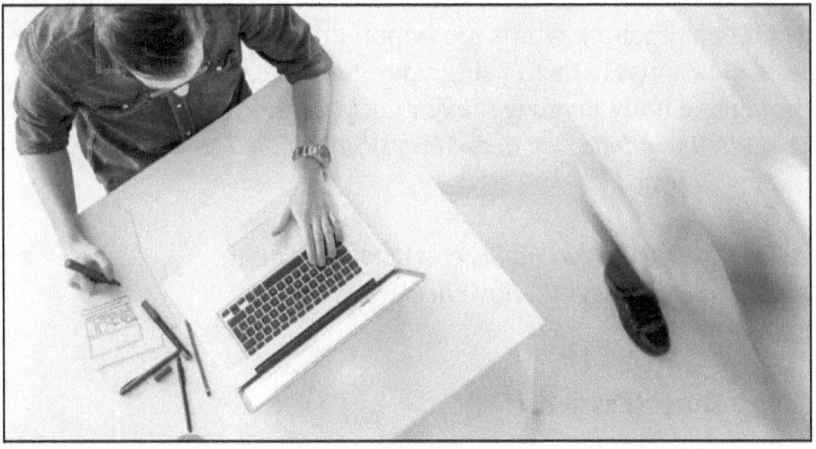

Stock Rocket

Staying in touch

Direction to a website can be valuable, especially if you have developed one of your own. Staying in touch can be helpful if new information arises. Your audience can sign up to this and you can add them to your mailer list with permission. Always allow them to unsubscribe as part of modern etiquette.

13 - Opening words

Instead of the hook you can use different styles to open your talk, but in the end your opening words are important. Bring the audience to attention and captivate them using your voice, facial expression of welcoming and body language revealing your motivation, (*see the earlier panel introduced by actor Mark Strong, hello! Makes you notice doesn't it?*).

'Hello, I am thrilled to be here.' (Personal/smile)
'It is a great privilege to have been invited.'
(more formal)

Telling a story. (Passionate)
'When asked to talk to the group I was unsure what subject might suit best. Given the fact I'm a few pounds over weight I thought I would share some ideas I've been following. The route to losing weight is not easy; not matter what anyone tells you...'

OR...
'No-one came out of Belsen fat!' Quotation. *'On the other hand being too thin creates the flip side of health risk. Take Karen Carpenter...'.*

Of course a picture of an emaciated person may not be appropriate so take care with your audience. Someone who is listening may themselves have lost someone to this disorder. The audience may relate emaciation adversely as an expression of cruelty, starvation and abuse. Back to your introduction –

Do not use –
'Good evening my name is Jane Smith and I am going to talk to you about Keeping Fit after Fifty.' It is too clichéd and the audience can read the slide.

"Hi, I'm Jane on behalf of my Health Club and hope some of you may find the material I have interesting."

Promotion is fine and helpful to the audience but leave it to the Chair if possible, your website, or any leaflets. In others words avoid wasting precious speaker time. However, use hooks like;

'Last year in the UK 300,000 people over the age of 50 died from heart disease. It is estimated that of those 300,000, 65% could have been helped by simple measures. We owe it to our family and the community to save the health service money by taking responsibility.'

You will also lose a golden moment with the audience if your introduction is bland. If it has sensation, and covers the reason for giving the talk, you will create attention. Let the person introducing say who you are. Provide your biography so that they don't have to make anything up. Once I am asked to give a talk, and have established the subject, I allow my mind to drift as to how I want to spin the subject.

What angle do I take? I want those key points to stand out and I look for 'hooks'. Hooks need to capture the audience's attention to engage them instantly and memorably. Typically, this is best at the start of the talk. When speaking to a professional group I had carefully selected a passage both for levity, a powerful message and complexity to meet the solution required. This passage came from a series of expressions Donald Rumsfeld; US Defence Secretary had used during the Iraqi war (2003) on 'Weapons of Mass Destruction'.

The feedback was actually positive and the comment came from a close friend as a throw away remark. It was feedback that I had not expected and hit the right note for the rest of my speech. The room did not fall apart but had resonated as part of the theme. Imagery works with oratory and can be of great value. Choosing the US flag was an easy solution as an image. I did not really need a picture of the statesman (Rumsfeld). There was no text though as this was delivered from memory and aided by a cue card.

Known things

'There are known knowns; there are things we know we know. We also know there are known unknowns; that is to say we know there are some things we do not know. But there are also unknown unknowns — the ones we don't know we don't know.'

I decided to learn the piece rather than put it onto a slide. Weeks before I had the text committed to memory but then I knew that I only had to juxta position one part of the phrase and the impact would be lost. My wife suggested that I read it out. Pride still held out until a week before. I copied it out onto a card. My wife reasoned that I knew it so well, the reading would sound normal as I had all the right inflexions.

The day was tense and I had a 30-minute slot. This was not a talk so much as a speech and I was dealing with some tough professional decisions. Up went the Stars and Stripes Flag and a picture of Donald Rumsfeld followed to cover the anticipated quotation without text. The card came up and I glanced from time to time but knew the passage well. Before I went further a voice at the front echoed...

'That's funny for you Dave.'

While the slide deck can be prepared as a story board, it is easy to have too many slides. You only need sufficient slides to tell a story. A slide will act as a trigger for your memory but there is a **rule** as far as TEXT slides go.

> USE NO MORE THAN FIVE POINTS PER SLIDE OR NO MORE THAN FIVE WORDS PER LINE

14 - Busy Slides

A busy slide is someone's way of saying - 'too much information' but the speaker fails to appreciate this is not only bad practice, but it has contradictory value. Options to allow the image or text to move around and in and out of the slide background (transitioning and animation) can improve but also lessen this effect. Used badly the options for Transitions and Animations as they are called can create one of the biggest distractors and instill annoyance for the audience.

The so called *busy slide* below is a demonstration slide to show how NOT TO. No audience will find this of value.

	Memorable points we need to discuss
<u>words</u> [*you see this, I think this*]	word – font size use only focus words use words to build on Bullets & animate lines (3-5) Don't read words
Increase audience resources	handouts conference brochure publication
Memory	mnemonics/cards/cue box/black-out
<u>**Image**</u>	Use image to help message clean, non pixelated, whole slide mix words-images Don't over animate
Finally	Structure, plan, time & practice allow time before conference

The five points below cover the slide above and avoid the problematical common flaws in slide design. By making a busy slide into separate chunks of information the audience will benefit more effectively by having information delivered palatably.

Five words

- Words
- Resources
- Memory
- Image
- Conclusion (finally)

Headings alone are used. When animation associated with PowerPoint is used the slide can be reformatted, given bullet headings reducing the titles to four instead of an optimum five options. No heading has been used as the speaker will use the slide as a recap after talking rather than in advance of what needs to be spoken. The black / blocker slide can be used before any discussion and then a bullet slide can follow to re-inforce the discussion. The speaker aims to associate the slide with something already mentioned to help the audience recall the key points being emphasised.

```
• Words
• Handouts
• Programme
• Publish
```

Text image (bulleted) is what the audience should see

How many slides?

This is not as easy to answer as a direct question. As many slides as required! There are limits however but it is easy to speak to a slide for over 5 minutes depending upon the narrative required. In his book, '*How to design TED worthy presentation slides*,' Akash Karia gives an example of 200 slides for an 18 minutes' presentation from Professor Larry Lessig. One sentence gave rise to three slides. Karia is positive that this worked because each slide provided a clearer picture for the audience. In many ways this slide falls between one slide every now and again and a video clip measured in frames per second. Video is permissible but should never dominate a slide presentation, let alone one designed as a short talk. In general, though if you talk for more than 30 seconds, move to a blocker slide as the visual value diminishes exponentially unless you can use the content.

Thirty slides for 10 minutes is usually too many, but if you create duplicate slides to show growth of some aspect of your talk, then 30 slides may be fine. An example of a complex diagram should be broken down into bite size segments so little chunks of information are delivered. Some slides may also show for 2-5 seconds if they serve a purpose. As a rule of thumb one slide per minute may be more than enough. Make sure that you do not use slides instead of the spoken words to deliver your talk. You might ask how can this happen? Well it is easy as some speakers find they have insufficient time and use text images in the belief that the audience will read these in lieu. This is an egregious error within planning. Never use a text slide to tell a story that you have no time allocation for!

Time needed to prepare

Don't be surprised how long talks take to prepare.

As far as the final stages of preparation are concerned, your title, subject, research, draft script, cue cards or cue slides should be near enough complete. The presentation might have taken 20 or more hours for a short talk. So far you might think you are already complete at this point but you have only created the foundation. Until PowerPoint has been correctly developed alongside the spoken word, completion has not been achieved. The last stage requires integrating all that preparation into a slide show. The slide show has to be delivered smoothly and appear effortless as if you had just walked in and talked off the top of your head. Only you know how long it has taken. Few people can take a subject and speak effectively in an ordered fashion as well as considering all elements of the subject unless of course they have given that talk previously.

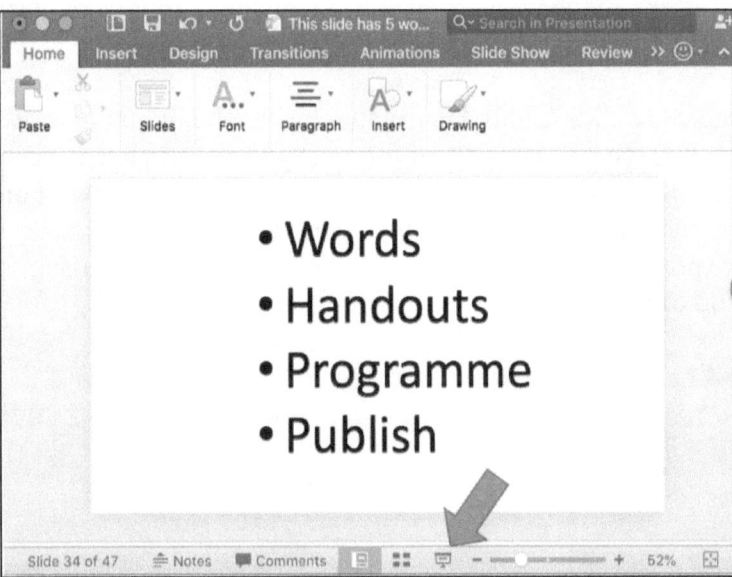

Making that first run

There may be a frisson of excitement, if not anticipation when you put the material together. That first run through will appear rough so expect this rather than disappointment. Select a quiet room. Using your laptop to enlarge the image to **'<u>slide show</u>'**. This is shown in the illustration on the previous page and is achieved by clicking on the icon at the bottom of the slide so that the picture alone will be visible. The picture marked Text Image (bulleted with the border is what your audience will see. Hit the return to shift to see the next slide in full expansion.

Some factors to ignore

For your first attempt do not worry about the time, just the order and the fit of spoken words (narrative). Ensure that your slide is relevant to the subject you intend to talk about. The use of a *blocker slide* is valuable. White maybe too bright and can distract, unless you need to illuminate a room.

Your preceding slide highlights the subject but should not give away the content. Once you have a feel for what you need to keep and what you might not, you then might want to refine your PowerPoint to ensure that the slides are clear when put to words. The blocker slides are points where you can talk and elaborate without using the distraction of a slide.

TRY ONLY TO USE SLIDES THAT HELP YOUR AUDIENCE UNDERSTAND THE DIRECTION YOU ARE WANTING TO TAKE THEM.

Avoid using a slide that is obvious

Consider the two slides below. Note the left hand slide 'Shutterstock' is a screen grab although in fact it is licensed under 'ProStockStudio' - Shutterstock. Make sure you use licensed illustrations rather than screen grabs. The example below[22] amplifies the point.

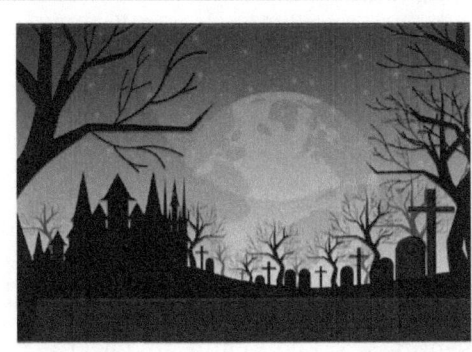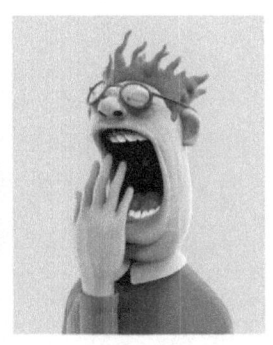

In the slide above, the left hand slide might suggest a graveyard at night. If you then say this is a graveyard as in graveyard shift as part of your delivery, this has a certain element of repetition and is obvious. The use of the right slide only can also suggest a 'graveyard shift', and yet is not obvious but expresses visually the effect of undertaking something late at night. To state graveyard shift without the graveyard, but use the snoozy man clipart, has a better relationship.

---

[22] Both slides are licensed; left 'Photoshop', right 'Mottive'

15 - Transitions & Animations

'DISTINCTLY SEPARATE SLIDES WITH CLUNKY TRANSITIONS ARE A GUARANTEED TURN OFF' - DAVID SOW

In this chapter I am going to stick to three instructional tips. These are

(1) the advantage of T&A,
(2) the disadvantage and
(3) examples of how they can be used.

It is important to ensure the image you show has optimum impact. PowerPoint offer ways of presenting text and picture images to tease the eye. It is important that your audience can see what they need and do not have to work hard to achieve this goal.

Along the top of the screen are two headings that can be selected; **'Transitions' and 'animations'.** Both can be used together or separately. See the icon bar below.

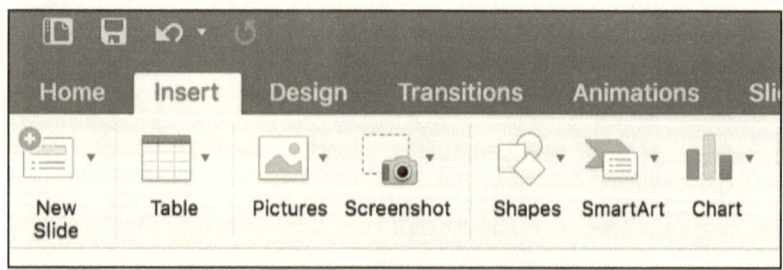

Transitions change the style of the slide delivery onto the screen. The usual expectation arises when your slide appears in the order that you intend it to. The standard delivery of a slide onto the screen arises after clicking and unfolds or just *appears* depending upon the instruction given. Usually there is no embellishment to a slide's appearance.

Animations change the order in which images within the slide appear for both text and pictures.

Transitions focus on the background while animations can alter any part of the image, including text.

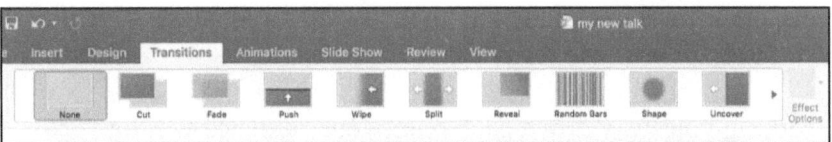

Transition bar

The icons provide an opportunity to design a dynamic change within your image. Perhaps the most useful options include *fade* and *wipe*. However, decisions are personal. You can in fact set the timing and apply short cuts. It is best not to become too obsessed to start with but always keep images as simple as possible.

Good points about transitions and animations

Audience attention lapse is a problem and there are many ways to interrupt this potential occurrence. Where carefully prepared, transitions and animations can be used to enhance the audience's attention to emphasise rather than confuse. The transition may do this alone by making the appearance of a slide enter onto the stage in a different way. *Sweeping in, roller blinding up or down, turning a page from one corner.*

You can keep the background stable and go to the image. When using animations, the image can fade in, then fade out on the next click. Animations can be set to a time period as *action runs*, but *faster action*[23] is better than slower action to avoid it becoming too painful to the audience. One of the best features relates to text and I use this for introductions, summaries and conclusions. Bulleted points can be arranged as a block, or one line at a time. The audiences' eye focuses only at the sentence in question. Chapter 16 deals with 'how to' in detail. If you had five headings your first heading will appear and provide you with an aid-memoire but also an opportunity to speak to one line without audience distraction. The second point can be added and then you speak to this. The original line can be faded in place so it bears a footprint, or it can disappear leaving the second line alone and then the third and so on. This is called *'Hide on next mouse click'*.

By working your way down each point your audience will be provided with a clearer impression of the headings related to the talk. Keep them hooked. If your headings appear as one block, the audience will focus away from the speaker, writing madly to ensure they record each heading and miss your words of wisdom.

> **TIP:** try to advise your audience what they might need to make a note of but also when they do not need to write anything down. This is good husbandry of material. Allow time for your audience to write.

---

[23] Italics used in the text indicates official PowerPoint terms used within the options available

Poor points about transitions and animations

A moving slide, that is the background, or the foreground moving around can be distracting. However, in contradiction, the movement you want is intended to distract. Why would you want to distract the audience? Distraction is more to do with overuse or improper use of the animations. Because images and text can *spin, splinter, radiate out*, these options may seem unique but not attractive to 'spice' up the slides. Animation on individual words can be most irritating. In this option text *creeps in* from one side (transition) and each letter follows like soldiers. The process is slow, pointless and has no added value. The illustration provides an idea how a name like my own could be used. The audience will sit wondering what the purpose of such a slide brings apart from the frustration of delay.

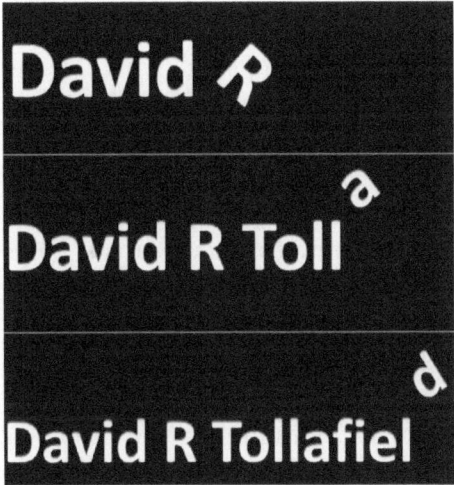

Using a method for no functional purpose spoils the smoothness within the talk by punctuating the delivery unnecessarily. Attention lapse returns if animations are over used.

Limit your use of transitions and animations

Try to limit your transitions and animations so any effect is optimised, but not used as an overkill. You can also copy to repeat slides, albeit slightly altered, to obtain the same effect. The use of transitions and animations lowers the slide numbers but if you attend a meeting and use older software, remember new features can fail if your attending centre has old software. Colours may also alter and all your hard efforts lead to disappointment.

Staying up to date with PowerPoint is not essential as newer software reads older software better than older software that can only read the versions before. All choices remain the Speaker's decision. To buy every new version is expensive and not necessarily that productive.

Messing around with slide designs is fun but it is important to be aggressive and remove anything that does not provide added value to the talk. Slide production from scratch can take a good proportion of preparation time, however a good slide deck does not remove your duty to the audience or prevent you developing your content for narration. Once you are more experienced you can cruise outside the areas marked as novice. However even experienced people are more at home with simpler options. My aim is to provide you with better control of your text slides.

DO practice and experiment to improve. When you go to your next talk as a delegate or audience member you may be surprised how many people fail to use the simple process of animating text. It may be fear of not being in control but criticisms about bullet points is well founded.

How to 'transition'

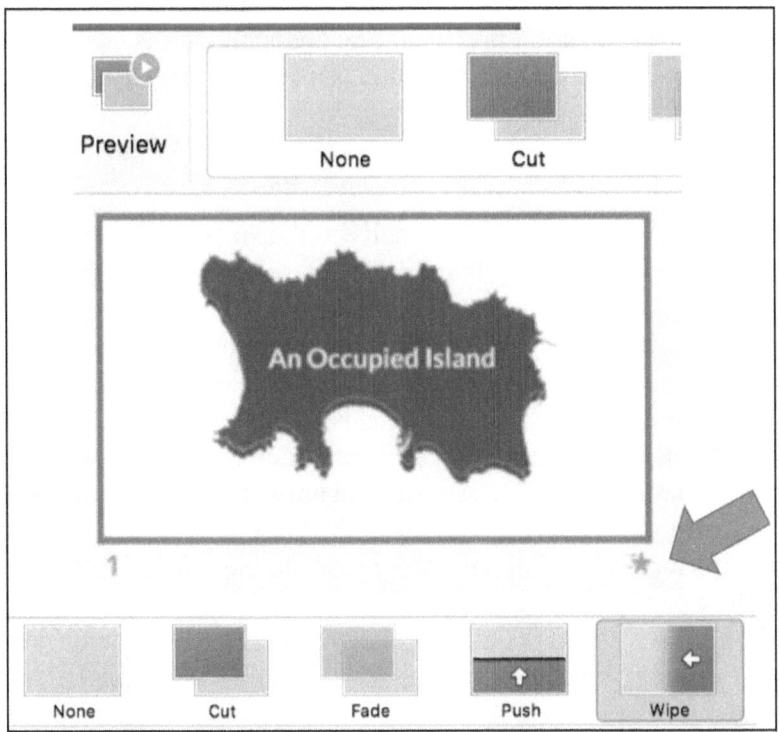

L.N.VectorPattern

The slide 'An Occupied Island' has a transition applied. The star icon, bottom right (see arrow), informs us that the slide has a transition. The slide has been numbered No.1.

'<u>Wipe</u>' has been used and the pane on the screen changes colour to show that it is active.

Top left you can see 'Preview' which allows you to select the slide (bold frame around slide 1 shown). If you wish to remove the wipe feature click on none or select another icon. The transitions operate on the previous slide so in fact what you are achieving is creating a blend between 2 slides. Done well this can be very effective.

How to 'animate'

Because the animation works internally to the slide you have to come away from the sorting feature (2) and open the slide up where you can edit it. This might sound complicated but think of the frame of the slide being influenced by transition movement and the boxes of text or pictures as being influenced by animation. Animation works on (1) but not on (2 or 3) as this is the slide viewer which is the view that the audience will see of the slide. The slide viewer (3) will allow you to see the features of both animation and transition.

The illustration shows three icons at the bottom of your PowerPoint screen but there are more icons to the left and right side. If you click on (1) the screen removes the side bar leaving the main slide for edit. And if you click on (2), this will also take you back to the main slide for editing.

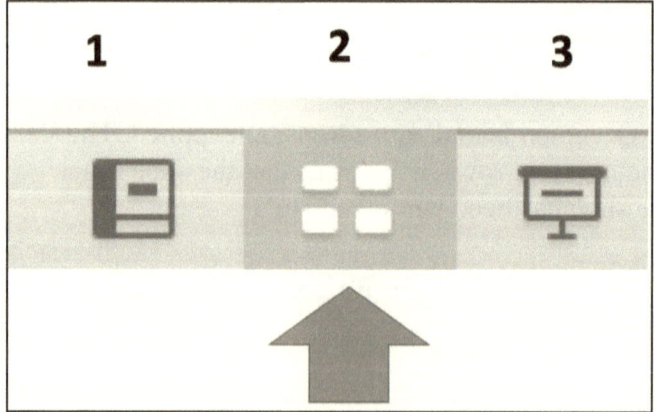

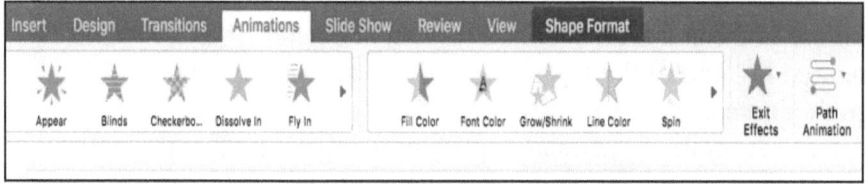

The animation features on the bar above are complicated by so many different options although those on the left are straight forward.

Animations

Appear	**Fill color**
Blinds	**Font color**
Checker box	**Grow/shrink**
Dissolve in	**Line color**
Fly in	**Spin**

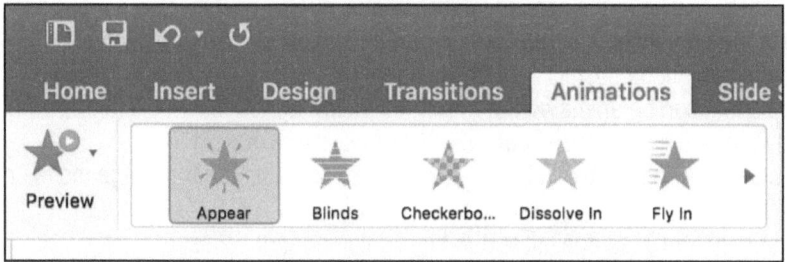

More options exist under animations but the key ones of value can be found above in the table (left side). The features in the pictures above apply to images and text.

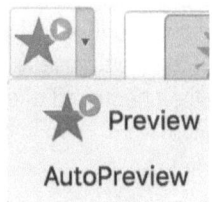

As before you can assign a feature to your slide and '**Preview**' icon as marked left end of the lower bar with the star sitting under '**home**'. You can experiment with different options to gain experience from the functional opportunities. Let's look at the bullet point animation in more detail in sequence 1 to 6.

Slide dynamics – more thoughts

1. I needed to show three newspaper publications on one slide. I used three separate free standing text boxes. Each box had a different date attribution. I used the spin method found in films where newspapers rotate. This provided pathos to the fact newspaper reports were significant. The use of the animations was to provide action, cover reports over 5 years without having to explain more than headline details and above all keeping the talk moving.

2. Using two images (side by side) as in an old building before and after renovation. One shows the original, the second, the change arising during construction. Sliding in the second image creates suspense if there is a clear gap visible to the audience as a transition. As an animation the use of growth and shrink effect might be useful.

3. Simple text can be animated but rather than allowing too much text at one time, the previous text can be faded out. NB *'Hide on next mouse click'*.

4. A picture of a light bulb can be given a burst appearance so the image moves as an action shot.

5. A star might be used against text to highlight important points.

6. When dealing with large text but you can blank most of it out to show the relevant section (Lincoln example). Either just use the section alone or fade out the background text overlaying the text you want to keep.

7. Another example of transition was where I wanted to show conflict caused by predators. The 'predator' character created by Stan Winston in the 1987 film was used and dissolved so the predator monster went from invisible, which was the point of the narrative, to visible. Having created this, I ditched it because it interfered with the narrative. However, I went onto use Dr Who's Tardis (a popular UK sci-fi TV show) in another talk with the chequered effect to show it transforming into the well known shape of a police box.

16- Text management for bullet points

The most valuable tool is animation of the so called bulleted points so that they emerge discretely without confusing or overwhelming your audience.

1   Select a slide that has a list as in the one below with five lines of no-more than five words. Shaped bullets (solid dots are shown) come in various designs. Keep bullet designs consistent throughout your slide deck.

- Ownership
- Invasion and acquisition
- Defence and castles
- Occupation WW2
- Current status

2   Select the green star **'appear'** with the slide programme fully expanded on your computer.

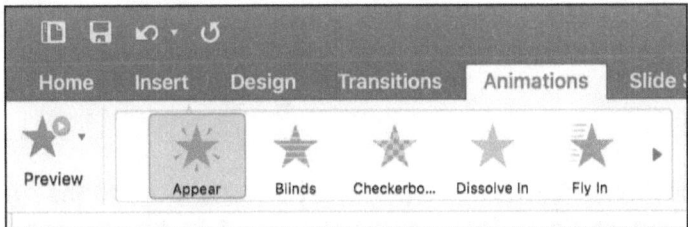

If you diminish the screen so it is smaller you may see the representation below showing an upward pointing arrow. The green star changes and just indicates **'Entrance effects'** whereas the box above is shown with the screen expanded fully. You will recall the traffic light style colours of red, white and green in the top left of the screen that allows the screen to be in two main sizes.

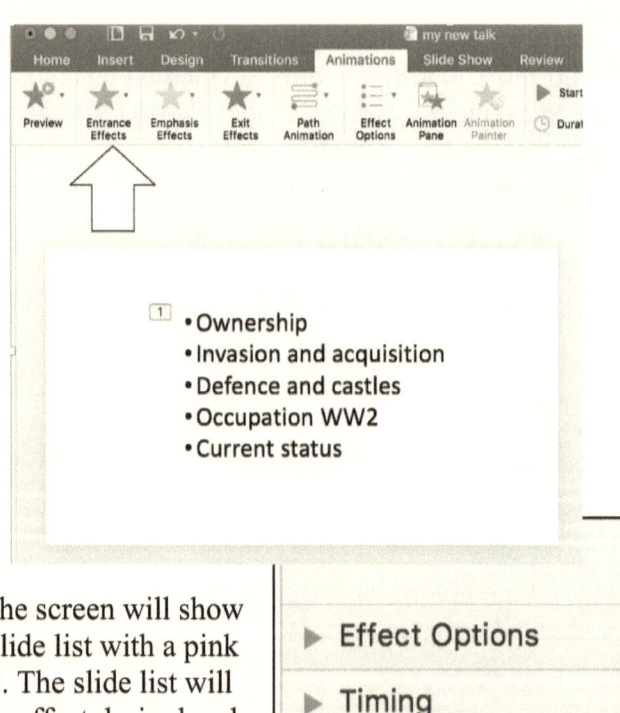

In either case the screen will show the emerging slide list with a pink box around [1]. The slide list will not produce the effect desired and allow each line to appear in sequence until you select the Text Animations.

3 The ANIMATIONS pane offers further options to the right of the slide. Select **'Text Animations'**. And note the drop down says 'all at once'

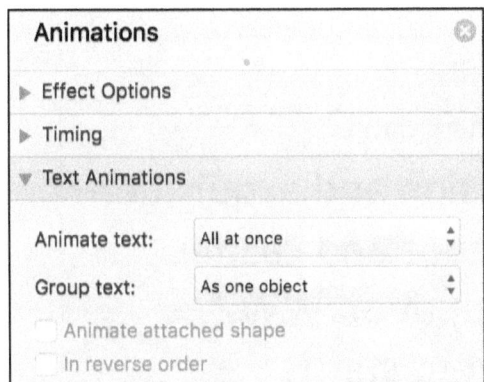

Leave the **<u>animate text</u>** *'all at once'* unaltered.

4 Select **'<u>Group text</u>'** and click the drop down bar until '1st level' appears removing as 'one object' and replacing it with **'1st level'**

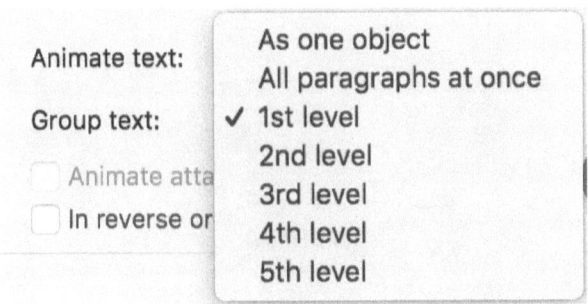

5 You will now see each line assigned a number one to five meaning that your sequential drop down will now work when you view this in the slide viewer.

1 • Ownership
2 • Invasion and acquisition
3 • Defence and castles
4 • Occupation WW2
5 • Current status

6 Go to the PowerPoint viewer to see the effect under **'Preview'** as shown again in this illustration. Each line of the list will drop down after the mouse or slide control is clicked providing you with control of each line. Try to speak before the line drops and use the line to reinforce what you have said. This is probably the best method of using a bullet designed slide and applying the 5:5 rule: five words OR five lines maximum. Now refer to the next section, disappearing text.

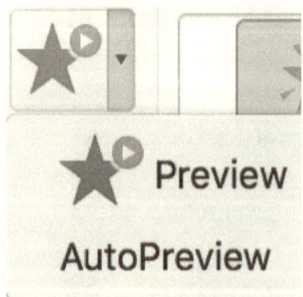

Preview

AutoPreview

Disappearing text

The illustration shows the slides descending sequentially.
PowerPoint offers the speaker even more control and if you select
'Effect Options' (page 107), under *animation*, then use **'Hide on
next mouse click'**, the preceding text line disappears, the audience
will only see one line at a time.

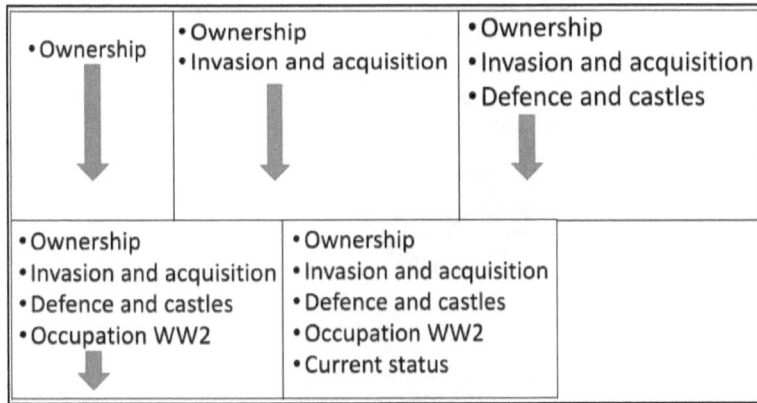

The frames in the illustration above show the growth of each
bulleted list. Here the lines build upon each other rather than
disappear on 'hide the mouse click'.

Therefore, this provides the speaker with two alternatives. To build
the list or to show one line at a time using the sequence above for
disappearing text.

Under **'Effect Options'** ignore the sound options; whooshing and
similar interruptions which are annoying.

Timing: there are three options; *start, duration* and *delay request.*
Again as a novice use 'on click' for start. Ignore duration and delay
request.

17 - Timing & Editing

THE BAD NEWS IS TIME FLIES. THE GOOD NEWS IS YOU'RE THE PILOT.
MICHAEL ATLSHULER

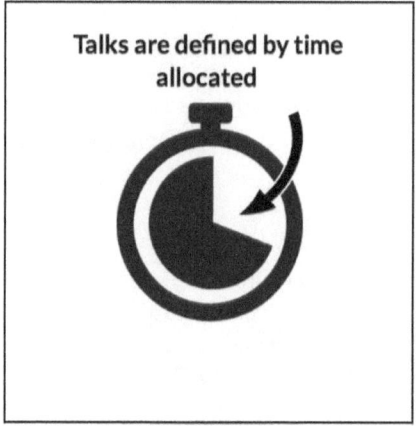

Mr Creative

There is nothing more frustrating then having to remove material you have become wedded to. All good speakers must be prepared to edit their content and ensure that any material left is relevant. Getting the material right is part of the equation that we all strive for. I cannot count the number of times I have created a great slide or worked on a great passage of oratory that is both apt and pithy only to find I do not have time in my talk. My talk is defined by the programme, the organiser and my audience. The key slots are defined and typically arise as 10,15,20,30 & 40 minute periods. Today most conferences and meetings prefer a 15-25-minute slot. A TED talk typically lasts up to18 minutes.

Slide show & practise

To locate rehearse timings use the icon within the bar which is brought up by clicking the PowerPoint tool called the '**slide show**'.

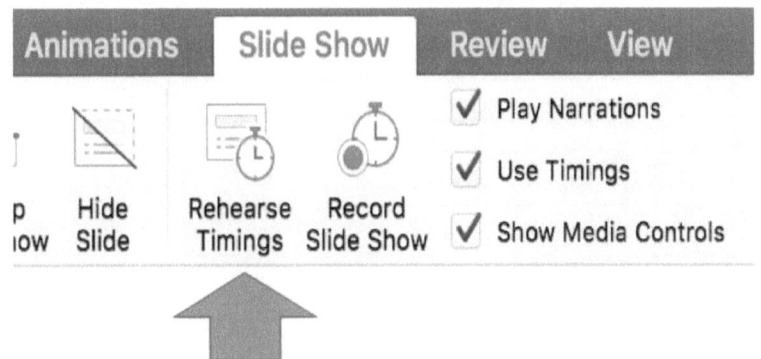

The '**<u>Rehearse Timings</u>**' icon is the best one to use as this allows you to fit your talk into the correct time period. When the time is too long (it is rarely too short) you can trim back manipulating the narrative and slides. Remember to remove the tick (shown) before your talk because the slides will run through on their own based on the timings you have practised in an auto mode. Additionally, if you record your voice, which you can do, then during your talk you will hear yourself. **SO DO** remove those ticked boxes; *play narrations, use timings, show media controls.*

At the end of the dummy run through you will be asked to save or not. If you save you can see each time allocated to the slide. You can now see where the talk was longest and shortest. There is only one caveat. The timing is not strictly accurate if compared to a stop watch or Smart phone timer. The time taken and recorded by PowerPoint slide show maybe slightly shorter. This may not be the case for newer packages than mine.

A scientific approach when speaking with slides

Example	Time (minutes)
Header	0.38
Slide 1	0.56
Slide 2	2.04
Slide 3	1.75
Slide 4	1.03
Slide 5	2.39
Slide 6	1.37
Slide 7	2.78
Slide 8	2.05
Slide 9	2.65

Total = 17.00 mins with an average slide time of 1.70 mins for a time period of 20 mins.

The **Custom Show** allows you to re-position any slides you want.

The Hide Slide allows the slide to remain within the show, but will not be visible when played in full monitor view. I would advise that you save your first edition and change the file name making it clear which version it is; alpha, beta, gamma etc. You can put a date on the file name or call it Version 1 or V.1.0 with the date 080318. This means should you suffer a mishap you have a version you can go back to, albeit with some inevitable loss of work.

Recording Slide Show is another useful facility allowing you to hear your voice. Initially this section will cover your dummy run and push you into self edit mode to trim back. We have already talked about timing but applying timing to practise is important if you want to polish your talk.

18 – Polishing Your Talk

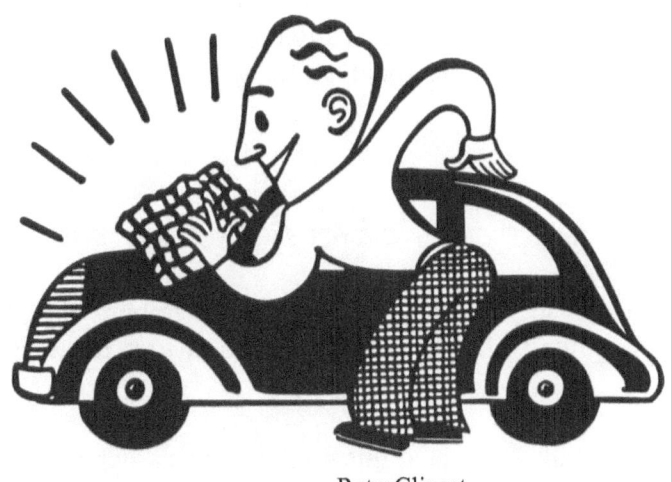

RetroClipart

There are two parts to the final polish.

Time honing
Fitting in the narrative

I have to admit I am never happy until I have feedback from an audience. There is always something to improve upon. You might leave parts you intended out, purely because of nerves and you had a memory lapse during the talk. The audience probably won't notice unless it was the main reason you gave your talk and found yourself wandering into the desert of speaking *too much* off the cuff.

Passion can run away with all of us causing us to lose rather than gain. Passion is important but it still needs controlling. You have to ensure timing is right first. The amount of material must fit into the allocated speaking slot. That material, the narrative, could sound stilted like a *Dalek* or sound as if you were quoting chunks of prose.

The important part of speaking is to sound natural and as if you were having a cosy chat. This means you must know what you want to say but should not try to learn what you need to say. The more natural your delivery the better. To achieve this accept that you may say the same thing in many different ways. It really doesn't matter as long as what you say fits, is relevant, clear and not rushed.

Time honing

ALLOW SUFFICIENT TIME BEFORE YOUR TALK TO PRACTISE.

This next section may seem overkill to some but the important part of preparing when giving a talk is to understand how to manage your time.

You must time your talk and repeat this until it comes down to the time required. It is best to aim shy of the target time so you have reserve.

Although in danger of repeating this advice, small informal talks are easier than formal talks with larger audiences. There is more latitude with the informal talk. Time allowances might be flexible, but please don't take unnecessary liberties. Remember your audience. They may not be as passionate as you are so do not squeeze more material in because you think they need to know everything there is to know.

To check your time, you can create a table. Either drawing by hand, or by using a word processor or spreadsheet. Along one side list the slide number. If you want, add the title of each slide. You can add notes if needed. The date of each attempt could also be useful if you want to examine the effect of lapses between individual practise runs. Do they appear around the same time or are they different? By how much does each time sequence vary? How close are you to achieving you aim?

Editing slides

While everyone copes with pressures in different ways, I would suggest that to leave your preparation until two weeks before is cutting it fine, especially if you need to trim and edit. If you leave planning until 2 weeks before the talk, then you are placing yourself in the red zone on the tachometer!

Example

Slide No. 1,2 etc
Name of slide (action).
Time recorded by PowerPoint

Data

1. Man walking dog   - 0.56 mins
2. Picture of car   -1.03 mins

... 3,4,5 etc

Add the times up:

Final time for talk   - 24.12 mins
Target for talk   - 20.00 mins
Trim back   - 4-5 minutes

Assuming that you work and have other commitments, and also have prepared much of the background four weeks before hand, you should find the timescale about right. You may still have a script to develop.

Even if you do not use a script much, it can help guide you and allow editing of narrative. Again, it is suggested that you don't try and learn the talk from a script as a novice. It is usually sufficient to learn the order and allow natural narrative to flow. Some like to speak to a mirror, or wall, into a dictaphone or have someone listen. Recruiting your partner or friend is a little onerous for them so it is best to devise a system for yourself. When running through your slides speak to the laptop or projector wall, or an imaginary audience. Try to practise speaking each day where possible to improve natural flow and to become accustomed to the order of the slides. The timings will adjust with your narrative. The narrative ideally uses the slide to reinforce your words, create interest, drive impact and help tell the story you wish to tell. Remember if you speak for too long to an image, go to a blocker slide. Let the narrative drive the slide not the other way around, except of course in the planning stage when you are using your slides as a story board in draft.

Fitting in the narrative

Title: Let us consider a fictional talk which borders on health. A fitness instructor desires to give a talk at her local gym, 'Nobbies', to interested senior members.
The title could be - 'Keeping Fit after Fifty'. The two *effs* make a good sound and the title is <u>short</u>.

Talk: Your talk covers the problems with modern society, its' impact on health and lack of exercise and you want to show how to modify the effects.

You will want to use data from your research about 'Health Town' and your own club called Nobbies Health Club, named after Norbert Clark a famous football player in Health Town.

Images: You have selected quality images of objects and people to make your point. You will need some text and this will be discreet. Not too much, just simple headings to guide your audience.

Time so far: Your target time has been missed by 4-5 mins (page 115). There are only three things you can do.

- Speed up your talking
- Cut out some narrative
- Cut out one or more slides

Speed up!

You should never speed up because your speaking voice must remain relaxed, clear and not slurred. Speaking quickly loses clarity, becomes stilted and boring. This gives the audience the impression – you are in a hurry.

Editing out

Remove material not required. You might have wanted to add in a survey that you had previously carried out on the cost of gyms and this took up 0.45mins speaking time. The detail and naming of each health centre, their individual prices. Remove it as you can shorten this to;

'Costs vary in the local area of Health town typically between £290 - £500.'

Remember in solo talks you can add information within the Question & Answer time, so leave material for later. You might not be able to do this in professional, multi-speaker talks.   In the situation where you might think the detail important, provide a handout or put up a graph - histographs are best at showing the data visually. Note that is it is better practise to keep to one point per slide rather than making the graph complex.

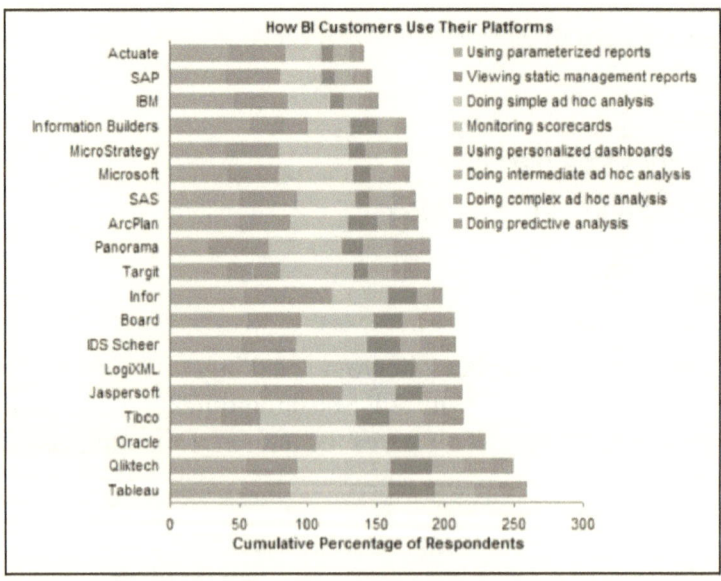

Source: https://venngage.com/blog/how-to-choose-the-best-charts-for-your-infographic/

The slide shown is very 'busy' and overlaps with different data. You would have to be into statistics to follow this type of presentation unless the speaker took a while to explain the material and the analysis.

Do not spend time talking about the graph intimately, only highlight the lowest cost to highest cost. If your talk is around economics of keeping fit, then you need to change your narrative. The data may be more important in this situation.

Cutting out slides?

There is a saying when writing. *'Prepare to kill your darlings!'* You have a picture of a man walking a dog. How important is this slide? Do you need it? Is there any other slide you see that could be trimmed back? Now this is where your table comes in as you can check trends. Where are the big fluctuations? Is your narrative too long? Do you keep adding more narrative?

TIP: If something is too intrusive chop it out. With the slide goes the narrative that is causing the problem. As we polish we can see if the narrative is also chunky and needs rewording or trimming.

Inspiration

A SUDDEN BURST OF CEREBRAL ENERGY THAT PROVIDES A NEW PERSPECTIVE

As you polish your talk there is some personal satisfaction in reaching the end of your journey. However, it is not unusual to have to make last minute changes. In fact, this is not unusual so accept the dilemma. The brain has been attuned to finding the best way to communicate your thoughts and although it is unlikely at this stage you will be re-writing the script, thoughts crystallise and last minute alterations now seem appropriate. There is nothing wrong with this and if you think your talk will be improved then I would go for it.

This has happened to me and I have very occasionally changed my mind during the presentation; without good planning this sudden flexibility will not work as you will also need to stay on track.

Connecting Slide to Narrative

'DON'T TRANSMIT, COMMUNICATE' - ERIC BERGMAN

Looking at the fictitious talk entitled **'Keeping Fit at Fifty',** a log of slide times identifies our performance. You may recognise some of this data from the section under scientific approach. The slides in the next example have been expanded. The log is useful and allows strategic manipulation of the slides. Hopefully at this stage, no matter the temptation try not to put any new slides in. All that happens is the talk will grow. Remove one or two only as an exchange, not an addition. You will have to calculate the average (mean) time by dividing the whole number (time) by the number of slides. Sometimes you will find one slide dominates. Slides 8 and 10 are the longest, slides 1 and 2 the shortest. The range is 0.38 - 2.78 mins which means you know which slides are costing more time.

Example	Mins
1. Header slide	0.38
2. Man walking dog	0.56
3. Racing track	2.04
4. Marathon race - people	1.75
5. Picture of car	1.03
6. Gym / treadmill	2.39
7. Blood pressure cuff	1.37
8. Hospital theatre	2.78
9. Coffin	2.05
10. Prevention methods	2.65

Total	17.00
Average time / slide	1.70
Time allocated	20.00
Reserve	03.00

Identifying the dominant slide can be beneficial. If you had a slide that took up 5-minutes it might be that this slide was the dominant slide and one you needed to practice with as content was critical and might be more complex. In a talk lasting 20 minutes you would need to trim your slides back. If you only needed one slide and that did the job - fine. It could be a data slide and much could be gained from this single slide. However, don't necessarily cram one slide with all of the information. It is better to make six slides from one, then introduce the data in small doses. This is more relevant when using graphs and charts. The keep fit example will be used together with discussion over slide design and size.

19 - Title Slide Design & Size

Having started with a title slide at the start of this book, we end with the same story. The opening title slide acts as an orientation slide. This slide can be left up whilst the talk is being introduced or you can move from this slide to the next one where the meat of the talk starts. However, your opener slide (primary or secondary) should connect with the audience. Their eyes will be focused first on the light of the image and then the words. Remove words and the audience will focus on you the speaker.

Keeping fit at 50

Jane Smith
Manager, Nobbies Fitness Club

The header or orientation slide with the title
'Keeping Fit at 50'

We have seen this header in an earlier example. The title was altered from 'fifty' originally written on the slide to '50' as it is easier to read. Compare this to Bergman's milestones analogy (page 55).

Check the spelling and capitals on slides as it is sometimes surprising how many talks given have spelling or typographical errors. The message this sends to the audience is; *cannot be bothered.*

Put your name (Jane Smith) under this in smaller letters. Use your own title - **Manager Nobbies Fitness Club**. If you work for yourself or someone with a brand, publicise this. The audience will relate this to the business side. Put a logo on or picture if you wish.

If your name is larger than the title you are saying *'I am more important than my title'*. Titles can be around font size 100 and the the Jane Smith name could be around font size 20-30. I often leave my name and qualifications off as the programme usually contains all that is required to meet speaker biography. The illustration used in the title figure is 138 main header and sub header / name 44 to fill the screen. By comparison look at the box below with relative font sizes and how much they fill the box. The larger the better is the general rule.

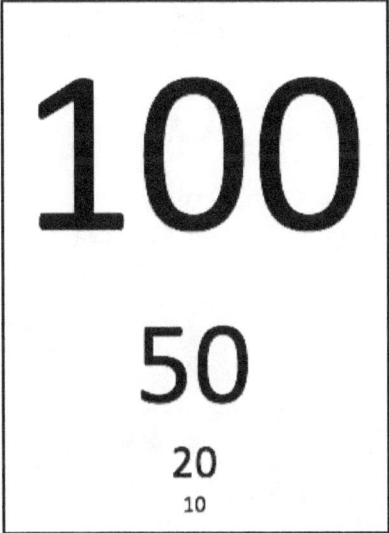

Tip: Avoid redundant space with text

Using illustrations

Put an illustration on if you wish to help provide the title with more punch. Remember the first slide sets you up as a speaker. Take time crafting it, but after you have carried out all the other preparation as your time is at a premium.

The option to use an illustrative picture with or without a logo is powerful and better than a header slide using text alone. Compare the two examples provided. A plain header and an illustrated header.

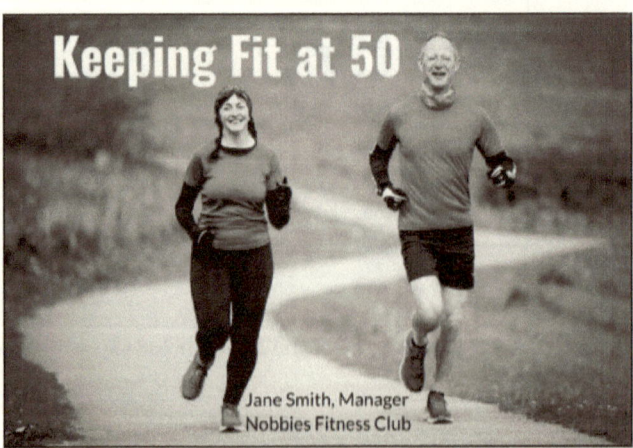

Steved_np3

The picture depicts senior adults which fits in with the talk objective covering 'Keeping Fit at 50'. The picture is licensed from a stock library. The focus is on *weight* and the value behind *running*. The title is offset to avoid cutting across the two runners.

The header is larger at the top, in white and not obscured. The Manager's name – for her position at the Nobbies Fitness Club is placed at the bottom and small in comparison so as not to overpower the slide. The audience will pick up on the subject quickly from the image and activity represented by the subjects.

Akash Karia provides good advice on the layout of the slide to optimise text and pictures. PowerPoint has a grid that can be overlaid across the slide so in effect the area is quartered. You can make use of the grid to layout text so it looks effect. The illustration shows a blank screen. You can see that the header slide for Keeping Fit was designed to avoid intrusive writing. The photo that you have imported can be placed off centre as required. To effect the grid as shown select 'View' along to uppermost bar between <u>edit</u> and <u>insert.</u> Select Guide and then guide again and division lines will appear.

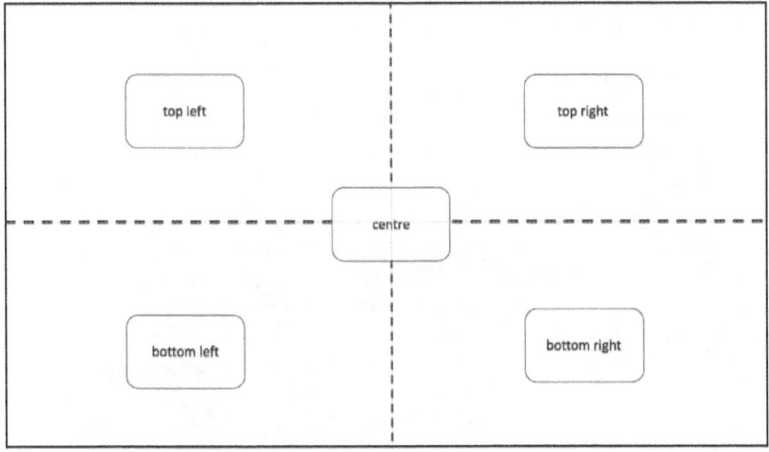

The rule of dividing a slide up allows you to use both horizontal and vertical aspects of the space available as well as use the slide's automatic alignment tool. In addition to these lines, as you move shapes around you can see if they align because dotted lines appear. Look at the next illustration to see the effect of dynamic guide lines.

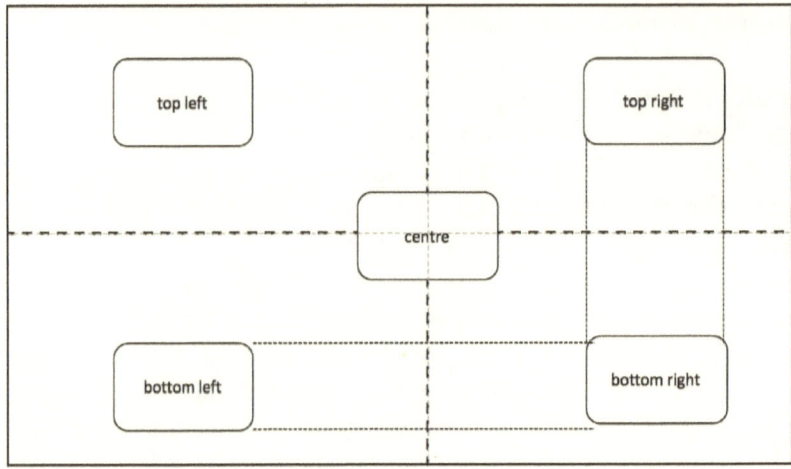

You do not have to select any icons or labels as this is automatic. The lines disappear once you take your hand off the cursor / mouse. Aligning accurately can make a difference to the look of your slide.

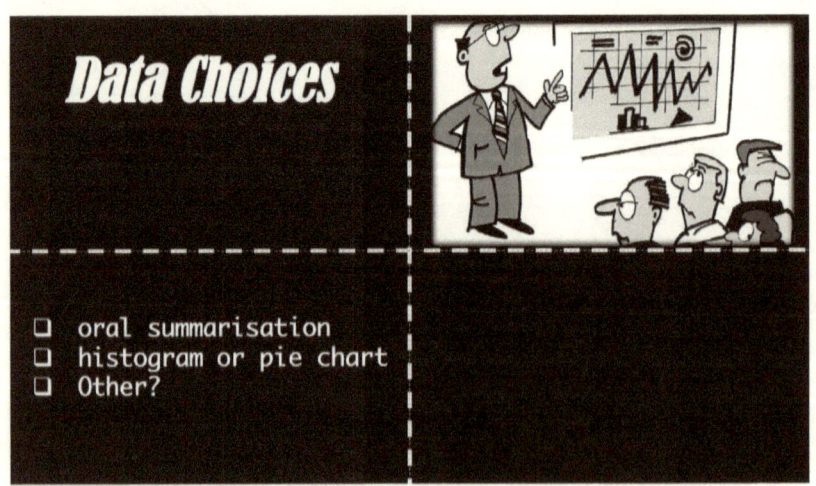

From 'This Slide Has Five Words'. Author 2020. Clipart - Alan Benge

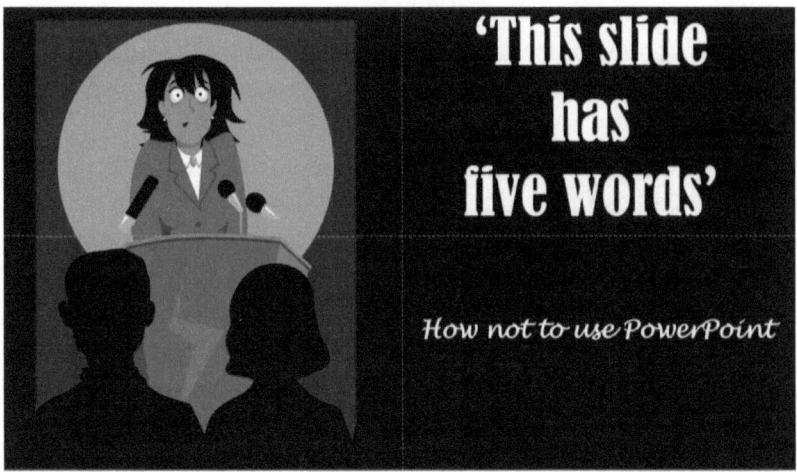

From *'This Slide Has Five Words'*. Author 2020. Clipart - Aleutie

As Karia points out, 'if you place points of interest in the intersections or along the lines your (picture) becomes more balanced and will enable a viewer of the image to interact more naturally.'

Thumb Nail

If the photo, or image is reduced to too small a size, then the clarity is lost and balance upset. The thumb nail picture and should be avoided.

Font style and size

The choice of fonts can be made more exciting rather than just using the standard Times Roman, Calibri, Arial etc. Not that these are poor font types, but they are a little common. As long as the style fits the subject; serious, comic, emphasis, then it does not matter. Styles should compliment each other and no-more than two font style per slide deck is sufficient. Of these two fonts, one might be larger with a need for the emphasis, while the second, or supplementary font can be smaller acting as an adjunct to the main font. Above the title (header slide) comes from my talk 'This Slide Has Five Words' and used two fonts. The smaller message emphasises that the talk is about PowerPoint and the clipart picture represents a novice speaker.

While it may appear obvious, those in an audience sitting at the back need to see as well as those at the front. The size of your font as much as the style has to be visible. The more words on a slide, the smaller the size. This is the reason for ensuring that a font is selected that is visible and dominates the slide effectively. I do not agree with all of Karia's examples as some of those examples selected are too fussy and the rule of five is broken. It must be accepted rules are to be broken in the name of making text and slides more exciting. Rotating text can be fun as it allows the eye to spot the change, but then the text must be an important part of the talk, one which should emphasise a key point. Repeating slide designs will lose their advantage and so as with animations and transitions keep the number of your creative slides down.

If you want to increase your slide variety, you can download new style fonts as well as creating images from the internet by searching. Searching for different options has never been easier as the breadth of material grows daily as often your search engine will find things before you have completed typing in the subject completely. Returning to the matter of the novice and kick starting your first PowerPoint slide talk, the latter has more than enough to keep you busy without becoming too distracted. We need to look a bit more closely at the narrative now.

20 - Examining the Narrative

Consider speaking to slides 2-5 in the 'Keeping Fit at 50' scenario, then compare these modifications.

Constructing slides 2 – 5

Use the slides as a cue.

#2 You can see a man walking his dog. This is good, both get exercise together and meet people.

#3 At the racetrack you can increase your loss in calories effectively. It is good to find a partner.

#4 when you enter a competition you know you have made it because not everyone can do marathons. The fact that you have medals is a reward for all of your effort.

#5 The motor car makes us lazy so we need to think how we can minimise car use. The other thing is we pump more CO into the air which ecologically speaking is not ideal.

I have deliberately made the narrative sound like a kindergarten book. However, the tone and pace can inadvertently sound monotonous. The task here is to remove and modify.

Modification

Use your slides but this time put the audience in the picture. A motor car can be used first and brought into focus with a picture of an office. Make this slide #2. The slide implies that the motor car is the prime choice of transport and therefore illustrates mobility, or does it? The office shows no movement - i.e sedentary status.

Communicate with the audience

Small group - go for direct interaction.
Large group consider giving options and approve the answer.
This is still interaction, keeps the story moving and make people think.
Use show of hands as an alternative method of communicating in the larger audience scenario.

Narrative examples

Small group

'When we look at this picture what do we see? Are there any similarities?' [verbal response]

Larger group

'Looking at the two pictures what messages are presented? How many think the pictures reflect the same message...'
'How many think the message is the same?' [physical response more likely] i.e show of hands

The two pictures actually represent no human movement or exercise which is where you want to drive the talk. Identify that people are limited in their capacity so what are the alternatives?

Pitch in with; *How many people die each year? And how many people have heart and circulatory disease?* You could offer up a multi choice question –

20,000 - 40,000 - 100,000

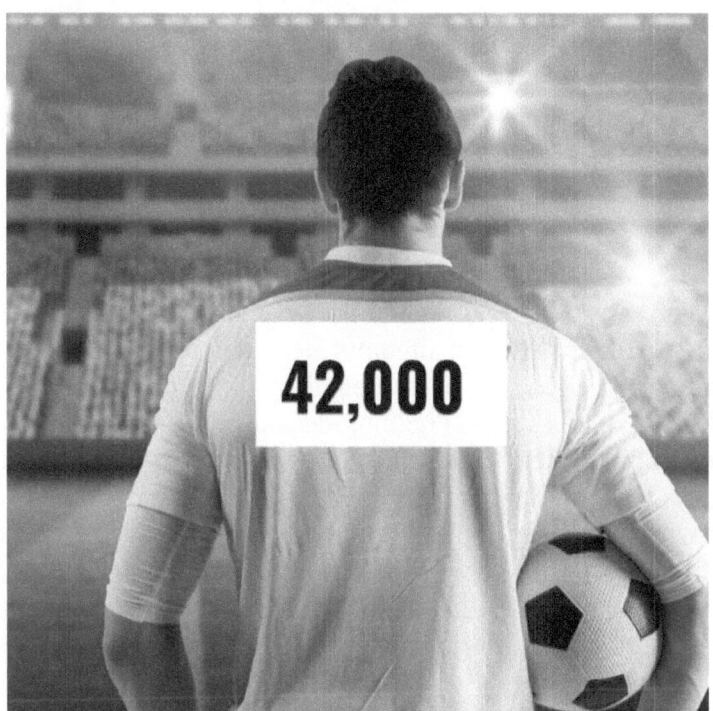

Wavebreakmedi. Slide #3

Slide#3 - shows a large number - percentage (70%) to make the point. It is quick. Take a footballer's back and paste a number onto the back. This does two things. You have added sports subliminally into your slide and provided the figure in a different, but interesting way.

'...The downside of course is injury can arise so fitness has to be built up carefully...' You can express information around more facts about knee, ankle, back injuries.

'While these facts and figures are interesting there is a difference between men and women when it comes to the effect of obesity and heart attacks...'

Develop along this theme so you add colour and dimension to the talk. People love facts and you can research these easily. Google search and find newspaper reports.

Slide #4 - Of course while we aspire to marathons maybe these are not always the safest places to look to lose weight. The number of deaths reported after marathon attempts mean you need to carefully consider your risk. Even non-obese people can succumb. It has been suggested that a runner called Pheidippides ran from Athens to Sparta and ran back after being turned down. This was 280 miles and took 4-5 days over challenging terrain. Allegedly the marathoner dropped down dead at the end! Although Pheidippides is associated with Marathon from which the name marathon (25 miles) arises, the sources and distortions from history contradict the evidence that the runner died, but it makes for good anecdote.

You might want to provide both sides of the argument for running with the audience, especially working with smaller groups. Engage different viewpoints but have research to back your answers and the direction you want to take.

Slide #5 is about right but again useful statistics covering air pollution and the need to minimise car use to promote activity contribute toward your themes.

Ask the audience *'What method could we employ to reduce car use?'*. It would seem reasonable to look at options such as car share, walking shorter distances, or even cycling. Is public transport an option? Slides can reflect some of these components but there are options for interaction. There are great opportunities to use some good slide designs.

Flipchart

Use a flipchart to write answers down so everyone can see the contributions as a group. A flipchart is usually a pad of A1 paper which can be turned up when the sheet is exhausted or the subject needs to change. At the end you could summarise using bullet like text to show the options on your visual slide.

- Car share
- Walking
- Cycling
- Using stairs over lifts
- Parking further away & walking
- Swimming

Your talk now has a clear focus on both the benefits of exercise and considers contradictory risks. Of course exercise is important, but it must be balanced against individual needs and that makes for a strong conclusion.

Nearly there

When designing a new talk, during the last week before your meeting, concentrate on trimming, editing and ensuring that the content flows. This is probably the most difficult part of the preparation.

Practise-practise-practise

Practise is important as time is creeping forward. Although I have created an example with a 3.00-minute reserve time this can change on the day if you get carried away. It is also easy to speak too quickly due to anxiety, which results in the talk actually shortening. Timing and practice allows a mental record of how long to speak. + 1-1.5 mins is not unreasonable and most session chairs will tolerate leeway in a conference session. In less formal occasions 5-10 minutes might be accepted, but always make clear how long you intend to speak for, don't leave it unspoken.

D-Day

The reality of your efforts now start to shine. Don't worry if you have self doubt, especially when performing with large groups or . with colleagues. There is always a sense of competition in the air. Doubt appears with those fears that you might have about your prospective performance. Let me assure you, if you have prepared - practised - and considered your presentation for your audience, the chance of failing is unlikely, even if you forget a few facts. Don't beat yourself up, chances are the audience would never know what was left out anyway.

Preparing Yourself

Waking early on the day of your talk due to growing anxiety is common if not normal. There is no right or wrong way so go through the talk one last time if you want to. Have a good breakfast, if you can.

Ensure you are alone if this helps; this is personal so you may prefer company of a friend or your partner. Exercise to keep you fresh and busy by going for a walk or use the gym, if this is an option. Ensure you have headache tablets. If you are staying away pack at least an extra shirt/top in case this is messed up at breakfast. Wear casual clothes at breakfast in case of mishaps.

Audi-visual check

Make sure you are early enough to check the audio-visual kit. Check out the room, then go to the lectern and make sure you are comfortable with any technical controls. Run through the slides where it is possible to check that no transfer changes have crept in that could lead to embarrassment. The transitions and animations are the place where most problems lie as well as audio or video clips.

Tip: Remove transitions and animations if you are in any doubt that these may fail. Additionally, use duplicate slides to avoid this same problem as duplication of slides with redacted text is a safer bet.

---

21 - Basic Artwork

Earlier I mentioned the value of *WordArt* (page 65) and how it can be used with discretion. We can use PowerPoint for much more if there is a need. Creating your own images is less expensive than using Stock photos and images called Clipart. Some artwork and photos are in fact free but the selection can be limited.

Clip Art

Imported pictures and images are considered. As one develops an interest in public speaking, the use of images becomes more attractive opening up different opportunities. Images can be humorous and based on cartoon style Clip Art.

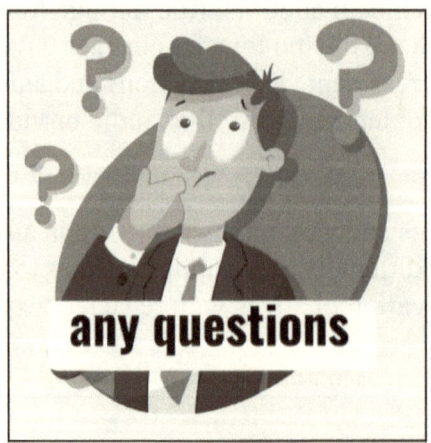

Alan Benge/Shutterstock.com

ClipArt is useful as it is non denominational, abstract from the reality 'real' people and may be used where the talk values humour.

Imagery helps concentrate your audiences' attention where you want it. Not everyone is creative and therefore using stock images and drawings will appeal to those with no intentions to draw. Stock sources are easy to find on the internet, although quality images require a license fee if you want to stay legitimate. If you are being paid to give a presentation, then you do require permission. Permission would apply if you capture people on your digital camera for use in public. Images can take a number of formats. Diagrams and lined drawings are good as they take up less memory. As you can imagine the more material you add, especially with colour photos, the more memory or data used. Free hand drawing certainly is growing in popularity with touch screen pencils. See the drawing of the crude man on page 138.

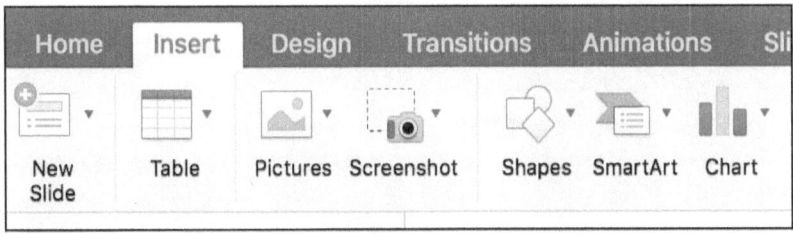

Select 'Home' or 'Insert' as both will bring up the **<u>'Shapes'</u>** icon

Free Style Drawing Icon

The picture over the page was created from the free form drawing icon that you can find by clicking shapes. It is the best method for retaining control. The mouse clicks on the wavy form line and you can draw with patience and practice. This offers an inexpensive method of drawing but it is not easy. I have used the method in some of my books and talks. With or without colour, line drawings can look effective and professional.

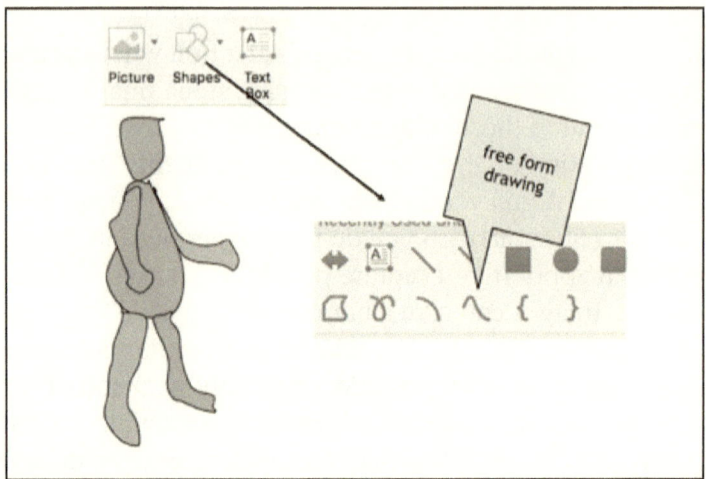

The crude drawing of a man illustrates that you can create basic figures, or with more effort you can make the illustrations more professional.

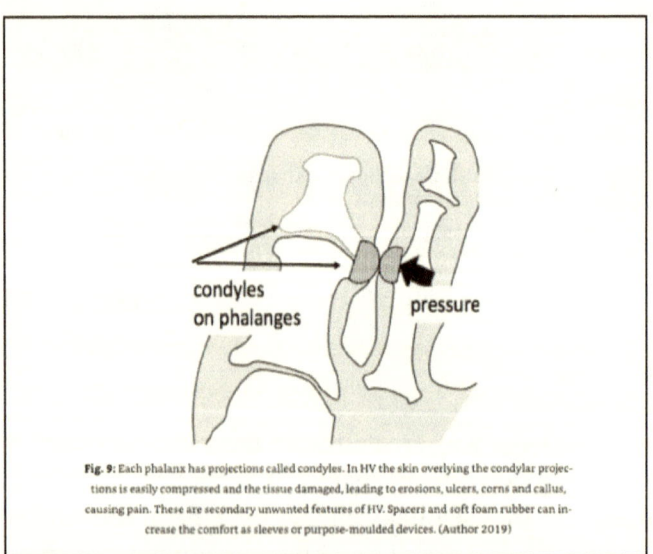

Fig. 9: Each phalanx has projections called condyles. In HV the skin overlying the condylar projections is easily compressed and the tissue damaged, leading to erosions, ulcers, corns and callus, causing pain. These are secondary unwanted features of HV. Spacers and soft foam rubber can increase the comfort as sleeves or purpose-moulded devices. (Author 2019)

The illustration above comes from a technical book using PowerPoint. (Tollafield 2019)

The illustration was created to show anatomical relationships as a medical illustration (author). PowerPoint drawing can be performed without the need to employ artists. Another example used a photo converted to a line drawing with colour infill for an article using PowerPoint. This can be helpful when photo images are too poor to use. See next under pixilated photos.

Drawings used with pixilated photos

When a photo[24] is too pixelated for use, a line drawing can improve the look and provide clearer lines.

Having an outline to start with is the most ideal way of creating symmetry and avoids copyright if you can change the picture a little so it has your own interpretation. The picture over the page is an example.

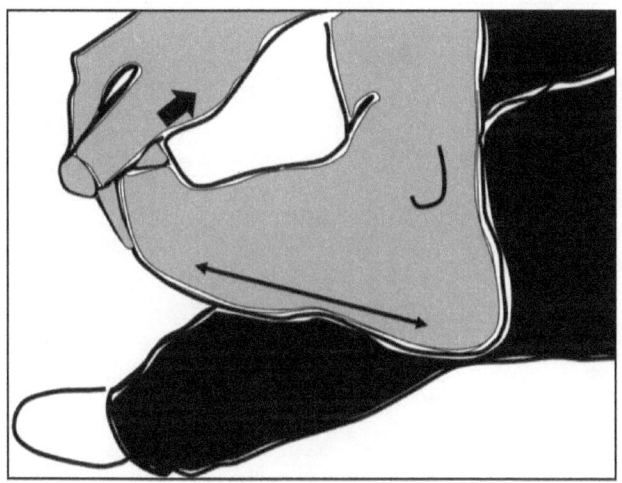

[24] The drawing came from a photo from Devrim Ozer (2015) Med. Bull. Haseki p297 DOI:104274/haseki.2479

Of course acknowledgement (see Footnote above) is also good etiquette by placing the origin of the photo/illustration on your slide in small writing, although this is not essential for most one off talks.

SmartArt

SmartArt offers a wealth of options and creates preformed drawings as circles, squares and hierarchy etc. The latter refers to methods of displaying data in much the same way as a family tree, but with shapes.

Relationships are referred to as headers and shapes. The SmartArt icon can be selected and a drop down menu will appear providing a selection of options. There are seven different groups.

LIST, PROCESS, CYCLE, HIERARCHY, RELATIONSHIP, AND MATRIX.

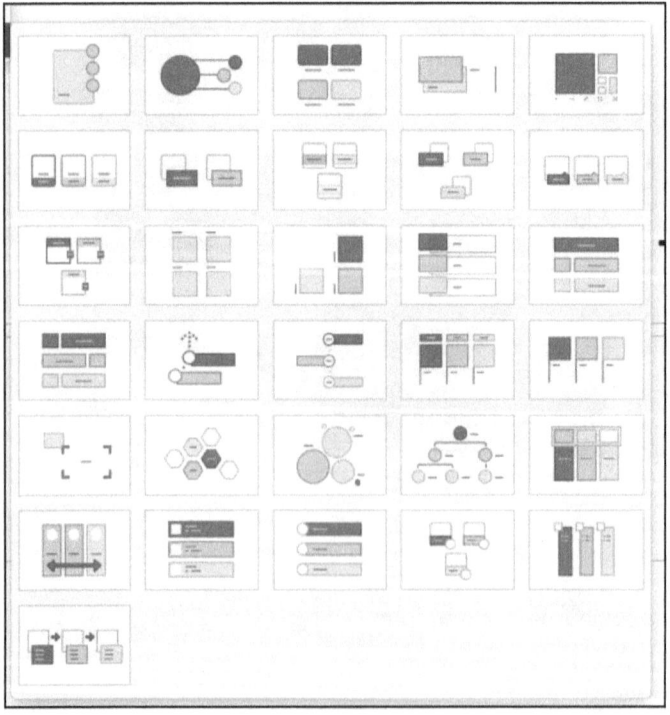

As an example I have selected 'relationships' and used three circles in connection with my *Jersey Island* talk. These can be used instead of bulleted points, benefitting from a visual image.

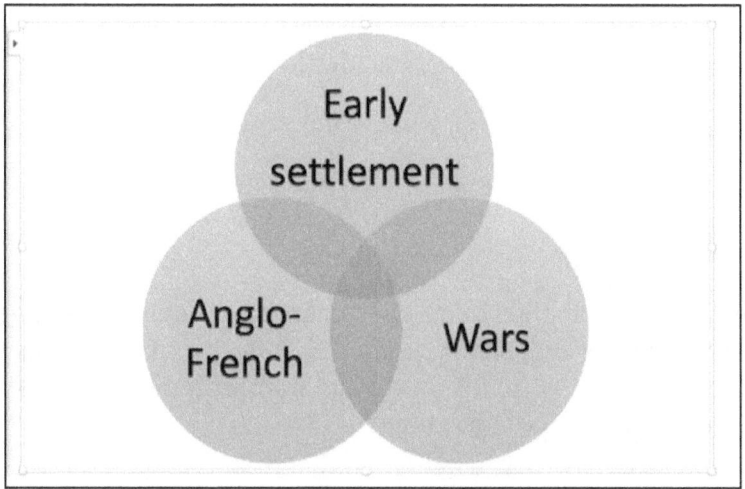

22 – Importing and sizing slides

Slide design is not just for artistic creation; Eric Bergman says,

'YOUR VISUAL AIDS SHOULD SUPPLEMENT YOUR STORY; NOT THE OTHER WAY AROUND.'

Importing

Importing is a term applied to internet technology implying taking a picture from outside and placing it into the slide. To carry out this function one has to acquire the image and transfer it. Do save it after altering the format so it can be stored.

We can use a screen capture or a prepared picture stored on our hard drive (inside the computer) or from and external source (outside the computer) such as a USB stick or flash drive, or external drive. Format types will vary although for the most part a format called JPEG is most frequently used.

Next we need to consider sizing our slide and the picture images within the slide. Consider the subject of screen capture (grab), covered later in this chapter 22.

Important Picture Icons

Slide images should reflect best quality, not appear blurred and should ideally be made large to fill the screen. Too many speakers use small images, often called thumb nails. In some cases, this is because by enlarging an existing poor quality image will cause it to pixelate or lose definition.

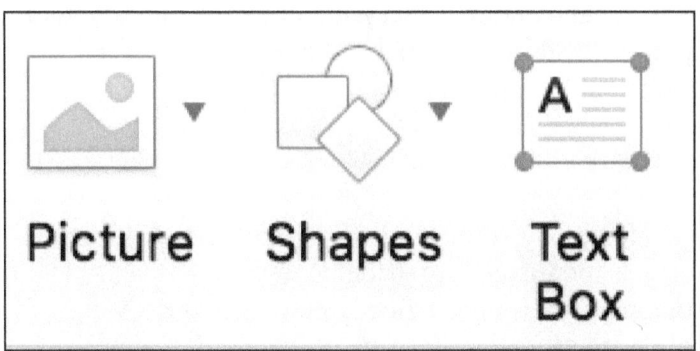

Pictures without text work best. Don't rely on text for your voice. Use the image to expand your oral narrative. So far much has been said about the many icons used within PowerPoint that when clicked make things happen to organise and design your slide. Images can be copied and pasted (inserted) into the slide. The left hand icon **'Picture'** is the one of several ways to import your image onto a slide. Find the *Picture* icon under **'Home'** or **'Insert'**. The *Picture* helps you import a photo onto your slide programme using a drop down menu of 2 options: **'photo browser'** or **'picture from file'**. Locate the image through either the browser or file to carry out the function of inserting the image you desire into the slide as shown in the image.

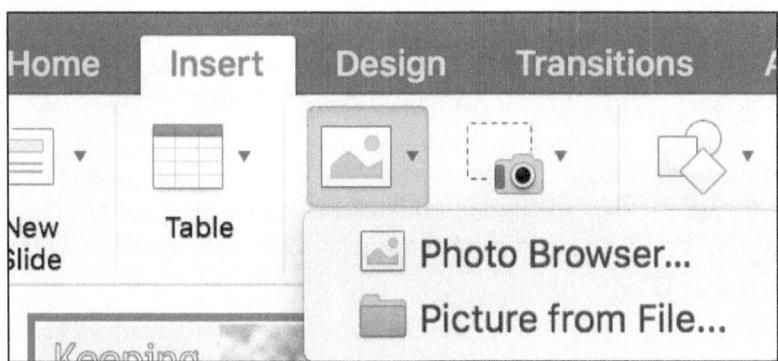

The '**Photo browser**' works via the photos you keep stored on your computer as dedicated photos. '**Picture from file**' allows you to locate any part of the drive, external and internal to copy across a picture stored from that medium.

Technical formats

Photographic images are stored in different formats. All formats deal with images and images are made up of pixels or cells. Too few pixels and the image is poorly defined. You need to know how much definition you need as well as how much storage data it will use. This knowledge can help you gauge how much quality is required as a minimum. 300 psi or pixels per sq. inch is considered appropriate, but you can achieve reasonable quality with less. An image can be manipulated into the best format before copying to a PowerPoint slide. Colour stability is important as well as compression size. TIFF is very good at retaining stability but for most of our daily needs, JPEG meet these demands.

Compressing data is all very well until the data is too small to be of value. If the data is too large and the colour quality increases the amount of data, then transfers are slow and unwieldy. Note a standard Smartphone prompts for small, medium or large quality. Large quality means more data and upload may be slower. I use screen shots in addition to stock photos and line drawings. To obtain the best quality photos use a high resolution digital camera in good light or stock licensed pictures. You may need to reduce the data if the image is presented in a format with a very large in capacity.

The following section might assist users of PowerPoint in respect of what image formats mean and how to relate to each method of saving images. The most common formats are GIF, PNG as well as, TIFF and JPEG.

JPEG (or JPG) stands for *Joint Photographic Experts Group* and came into being around 1992. This is the most common image format used by digital cameras and other photographic image capture devices and used for storing and transmitting photographic images by internet. The loss of quality of the picture is minimised and the sizes of data used manageable.

GIF stands for *Graphics Interchange Format*. It is useful for animations but less suitable for reproducing colour photographs but it is well-suited for simpler images such as graphics or logos with solid areas of colour.

PNG stands for *Portable Network Graphics*.
A key drawback of PNG is that it compresses digital images at a larger file size compared to JPEG standard which achieves a smaller file size than a PNG for a relatively similar image quality and resolution. PNG files offer better compression and a reduced file size compared to GIF. PNG is a good choice for storing line drawings, text, and iconic graphics at a small file size.

TIFF stands for *tagged image format file* and used for high-quality graphics. They are versatile and deal well with colour ranges.
TIFF is a good choice for archiving images when detail must be preserved and file size is not a consideration.
Vector graphics are mainly used today in the context of two-dimensional computer graphics and can be uploaded to online databases for other designers to download and manipulate, speeding up the creative process.

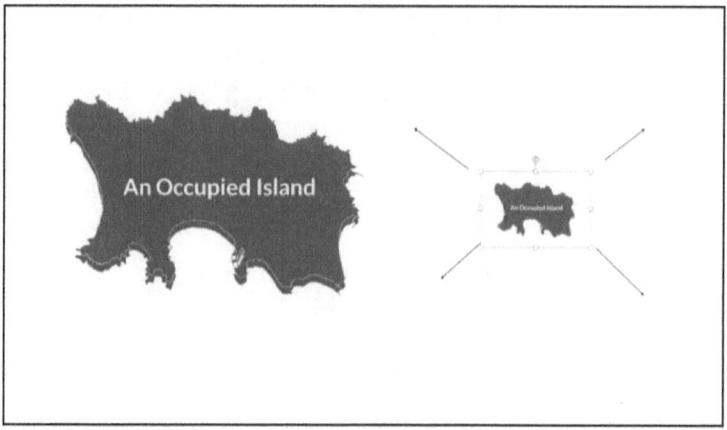

Sizing images

The image should fit the whole screen wherever possible. Enlargement arises by grabbing the corner of the picture and expanding the image until it fills the whole screen. The larger the better. The resizing bars are shown alongside the crop bars (also page 149).

Do not worry if your picture overlaps the outside of the slide; no-one will notice this when viewed on PowerPoint screen. In the figure above the left slide fills the screen while the right side shows the original size.

At the bottom of the screen a grey bar shows a sizing bar which slides to expand the slide screen, but not the internal components of the image.

The figure provided along the bar shows a value representing the percentage size. The bar reads 130%, while the centre of the bar represents 100%. To the right of the value [130%] an expansion icon with four arrows facing from the centre outwards within a box is a default. If you click the box after changing the size at any time it returns to (defaults) the original size i.e 100%.

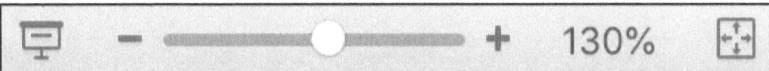

The icon to the left is the PowerPoint slide viewer that we have met before. The whole screen expands to show your image without any peripheral material and is how your slide will look to the audience. If the imported image fills the screen it looks powerful and very professional. Once you discover this method you will be persuaded to optimise your images forever.

Paired slides

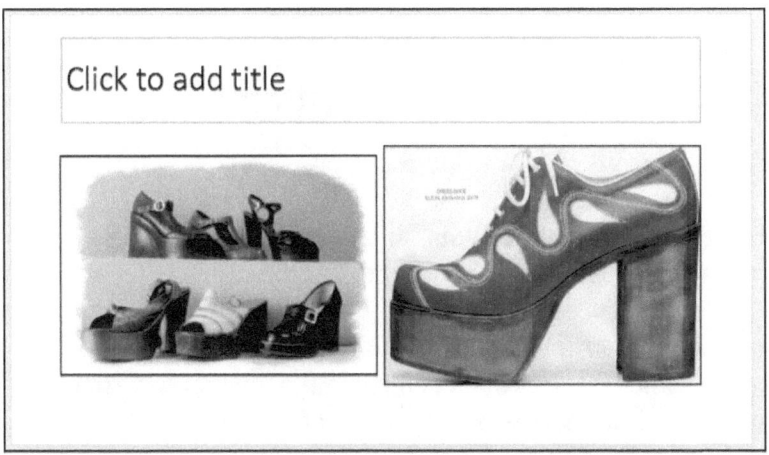

You may feel that you want two photos side by side to contrast different stages or points in time. This may be a picture of a tree in summer and then again in winter. You can crop your picture to size which is similar to taking scissors to the picture and shaping it to size. Symmetry is important so make them the same size to fill the screen. You can use two independent text boxes or a blank pane with two formats called click to add title / click to add text. Within the box is an icon with the 'picture' feature. The example above shows two sets of shoes. The title has not been added which is a box in its own right.

Cropping images

There comes a time when you want to control what is seen. Part of the image may be supplementary to requirement and so slimming it down is a good idea to reveal what you require. After this has been undertaken you can enlarge the picture without pixilation.

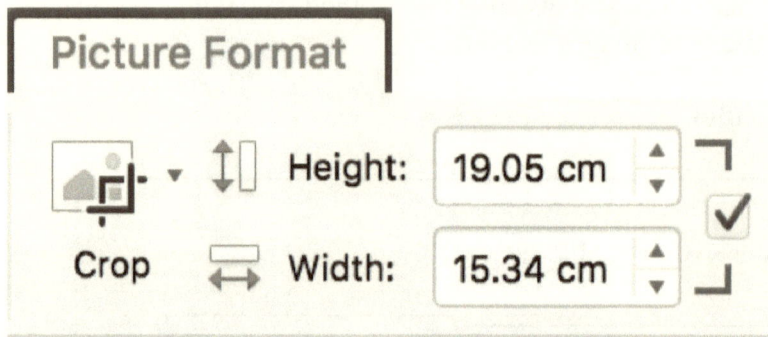

Once the desired image is on your slide, click **'home'** and then **'picture format'** will appear highlighted to the right on the icon bar.

The sign-post picture format does not reside over the **'crop icon'** and *resizing table*; this has been contrived for this book. Cropping works by controlling bars which appear when the crop tool is activated by single clicking. There is a distinction between the re-sizing bars and crop bars.

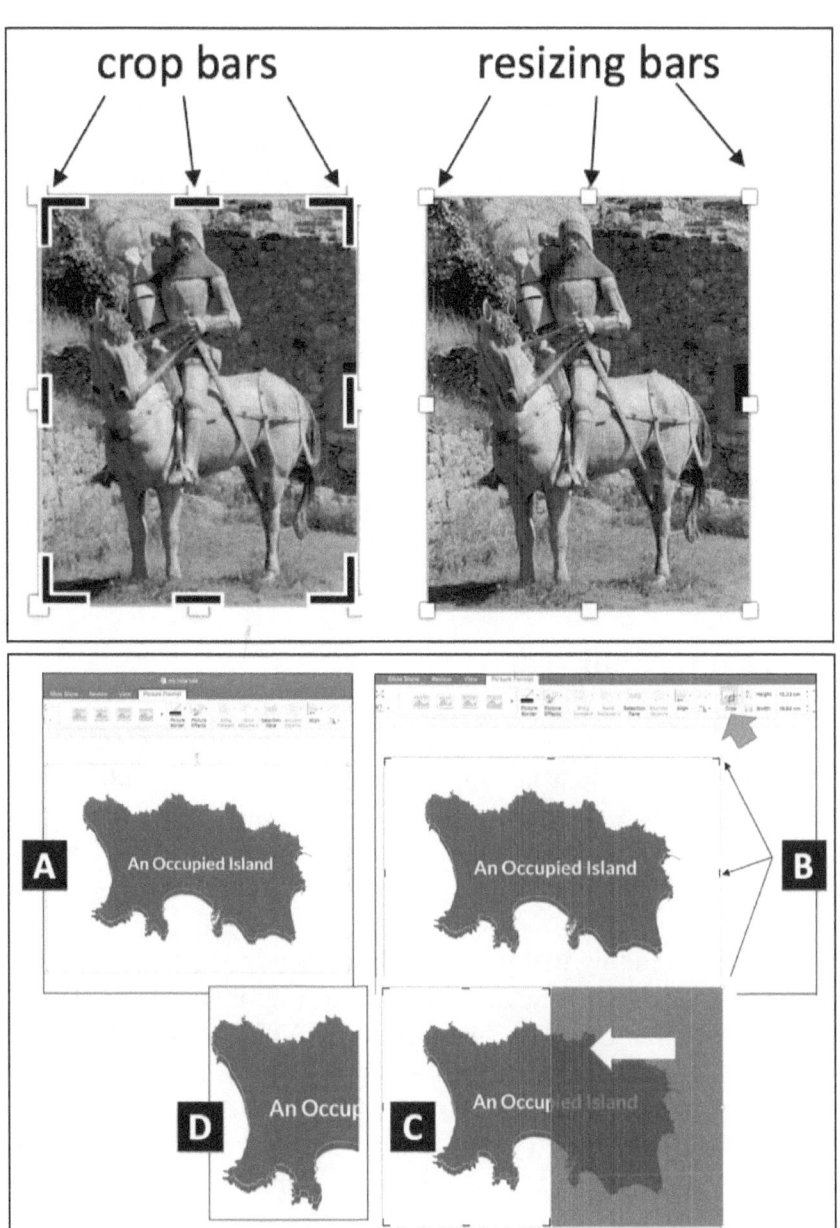

Click on the picture e.g (A) and the crop bar will appear, also indicated with an arrow. To the side you will see a sizing scale in cm. to resize the vertical and horizontal dimensions. This can be used instead of the resizing handles. You can alter the dimensions or use grab handles as in (B). The arrows show the right hand side only.

If you push or slide the middle grab handle, over as in (B), the screen will darken (C) and this will lead to the picture losing the right hand side and only show the writing i.e **'An Occup'** as in (D). By manipulating the grab handles the size can be changed in both horizontal or vertical directions.
To make the picture as in (D) larger again, grab the handles, achieved by clicking the mouse so it disengages the darker grab bars at the corners and sides. Resizing then is the same as it was for the enlargement illustration of the Island of Jersey.

Screen captures or screen grabs

These are captured pictures or figures from a computer screen. The most common example is taking something from the internet. Different computers PC or Mac have different ways of achieving a screen capture so I would recommend using a search engine (*e.g Bing, Google*) for the method for your particular computer.

It is worthwhile adding that you can take screen captures from your i-pad, tablet, or Smartphone and transfer this into PowerPoint. The brilliant part of this facility is that it is quick. You can e-mail yourself or sync into a *cloud storage*[25] and download. The picture imports into your slide so that you can manipulate the photo size but not the data capacity. I will deal with data capacity later as it is important to understand the problems when transferring data (page 168).

---

[25] Cloud storage was mentioned earlier as a storage medium to retrieve your data from any computer via the internet

The following stages **1-6** explains how to undertake a screen capture then deal with the image ready for use as a PowerPoint image.

1   Select an image from the internet. The example given is a recipe from an advert[26]

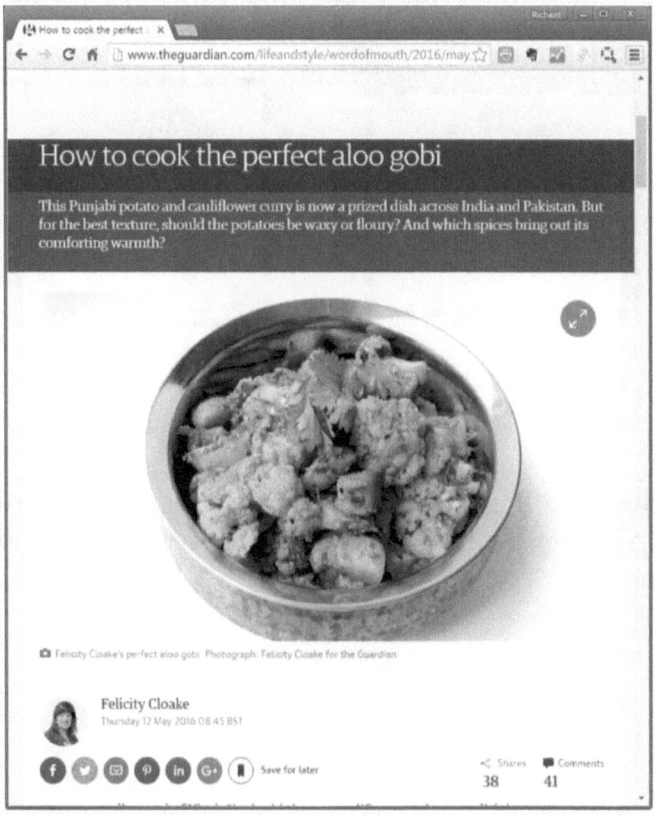

[26] Aloo Gobi c/o theguardian.com Felicity Cloake 2016

2 Place your screen capture bar around the part of the image you wish to copy. This is represented by a hashed border although in reality the box you will see on your computer may not have broken lines but a solid box line.

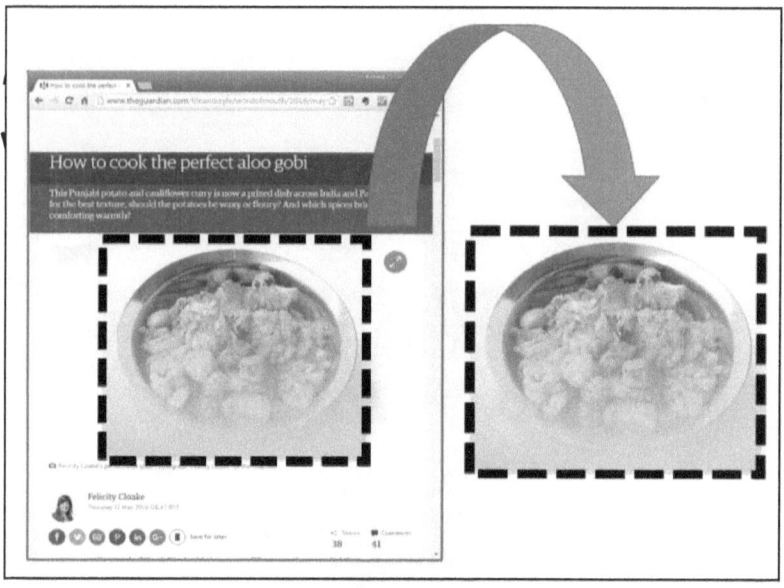

Now click and the image will appear relocated to your desktop screen. This is shown together with an untitled folder underneath.

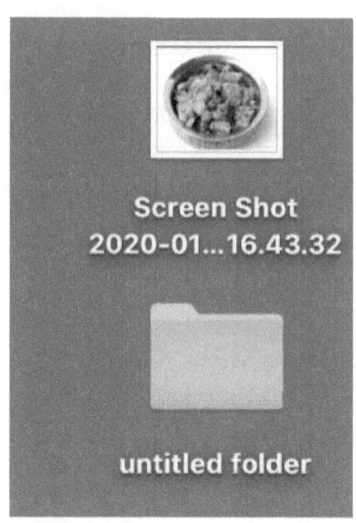

**Screen Shot
2020-01...16.43.32**

untitled folder

3 Click on your image called a screen shot labelled *2020-01-16 at 16.43.32*. This code changes for each screen shot and is unique.

4 Click the header bar with **'File'** and a menu will drop.

File	Edit	View	Go	Tools	Window

New from Clipboard	⌘N
Open...	⌘O
Open Recent	▶
Close Window	⌘W
Close Selected Image	⇧⌘W
Save	⌘S
Duplicate	⇧⌘S
Rename...	
Move To...	
Export...	
Export as PDF...	
Share	▶
Revert To	▶

5 Select 'Export' on the drop down menu. Your image now will be assigned a format and you have more control. Note that the code is the same as it is under [3].

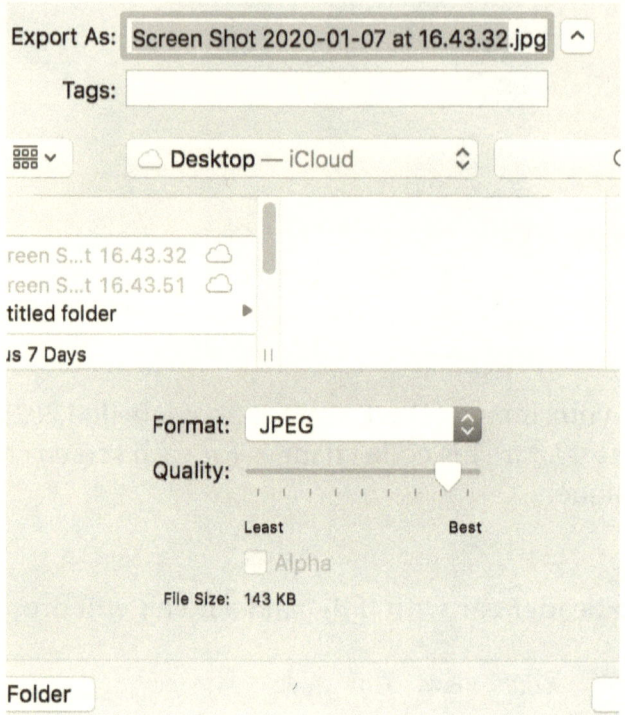

The top label states **'Export as:'** and is assigned a name screen shot 2020-01-07 at 16.43.32.jpg. The 16.43 means this was captured after the previous image (4).

The end stem .jpg (or jpeg) was assigned when the image was created. The **'format:'** states JPEG but was changed from PNG as this had larger data size. The **'File Size'** now states 143KB (1000KB=1MB, or megabyte). This is very small in data terms. The **'Quality'** of the image can be changed using the quality slide bar; i.e *Least to Best* (as above).

6 Now import the image saved on your desktop directly onto your slide deck.

Click on [Insert – pictures] or click on the image [copy].

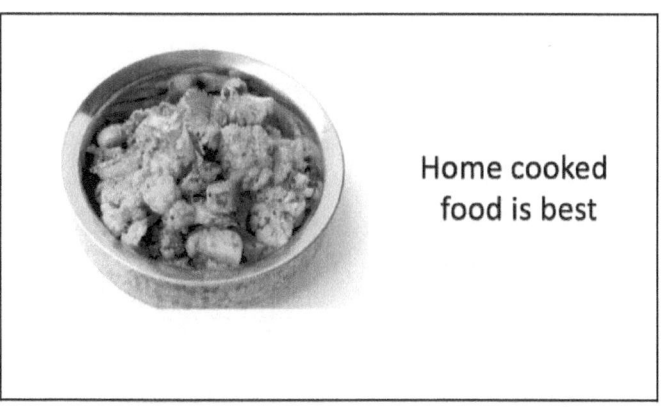

Home cooked
food is best

You now have a clean image of food with a 5 worded header and all set for a talk on cuisine.

Colour

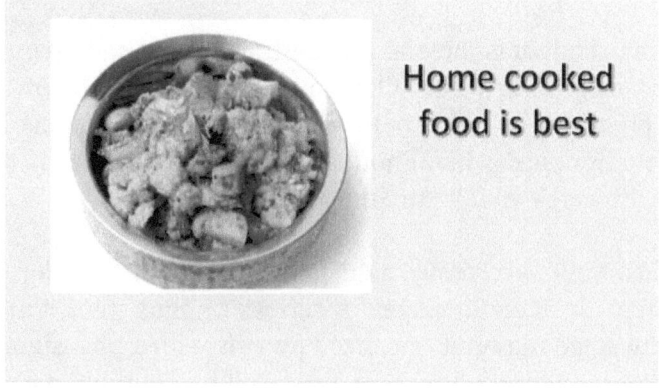

Home cooked
food is best

The slide deck now shows an image with a background (despite this book being in black and white). A WordArt title has been added. The background colour actually used is a light blue. A border exists around the food. To remove this border, select **'Picture Format'** as previously by clicking on the slide image.

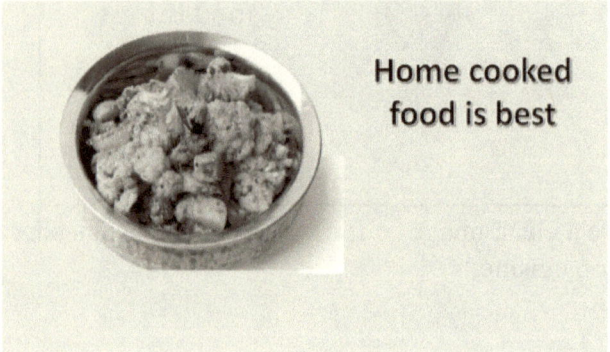

The far left icon shown is the one required, **'Remove background'**. The remove background is very clever and can remove a lot of clutter with photos. This is a benefit you often have to consider by upgrading to programmes like Photo shop. If you are a serious image manipulator, PowerPoint is really only a capable fill-in.

Follow the instructions to remove the magenta coloured border seen on the screen to clean up the edges. A series of minus signs will redact the unwanted material or resize upwards with a plus sign. The method can take a while as you take away and find another part of the unwanted image appears. As a quick and dirty method the process works well enough.

The options to change are wide with many variations. Graduated colours and shaded infill can be created. For most people all these options will not be required. The word format really just means adding a process to change something. In this next case formatting the background colour is important so it adapts kindly to the audience' eye.

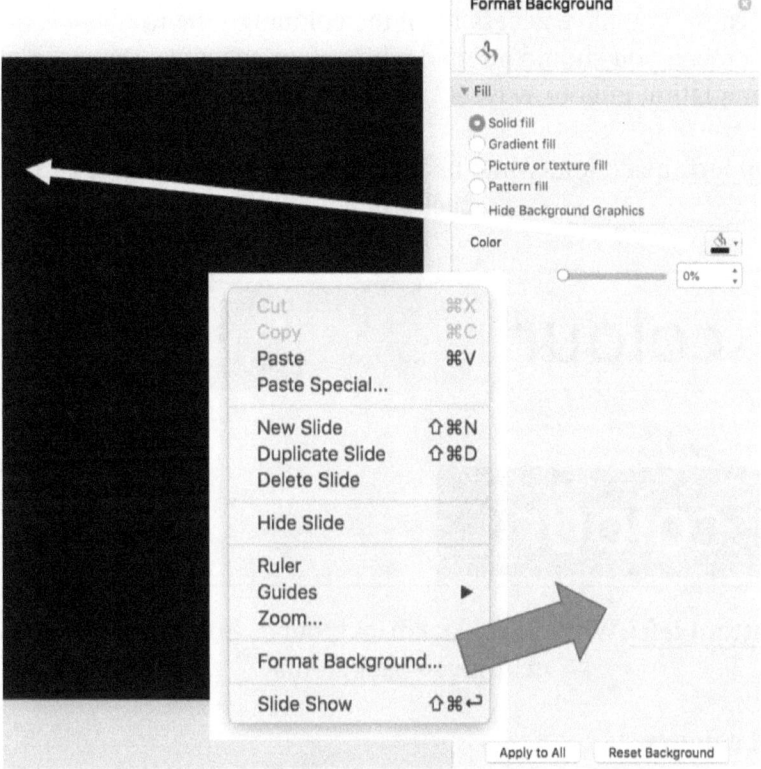

'Format background' is one of a number of options as can be seen from the two menus below.

An image needs to stand out but not detract from the story. PowerPoint will allow solid colours and graduated (gradient) colours for the background. As a rule, a lighter background is best so you can use white, very pale green, cream and light blues make gentle backgrounds. Shapes and outlines can be more vivid and stand out.

Solid or bold red writing on dark backgrounds will cause eye strain. Just because you have access to all the colours of the rainbow doesn't mean you should go mad with colour schemes. PowerPoint puts temptation in your way.

Top left: black text/white background. Top right: blue text/red background

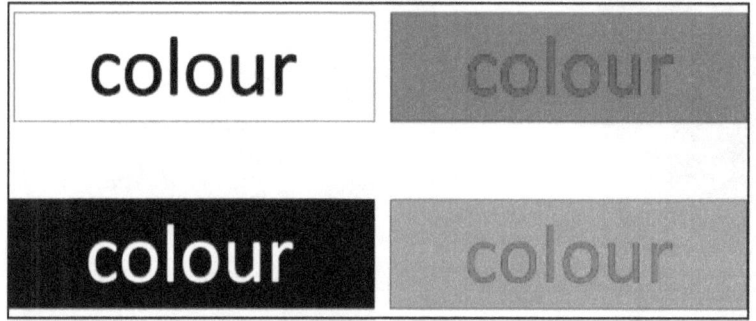

Bottom left: White text/black background. Bottom right: Red text/green background

Mixed colours

Although previously mentioned earlier, colours mixed up without a central theme can cause eye concentration problems. Good colour consistency will re-enforce the slide. Use strong colours for emphasis.

Dark coloured shapes against a light background work well. The use of dual or gradient filled colours, textures, shadows, reflections, glow, soft edges and more can be manipulated but such detail is not required in this manual intended as it us only as an introduction to PowerPoint and the basic peformance.

Design

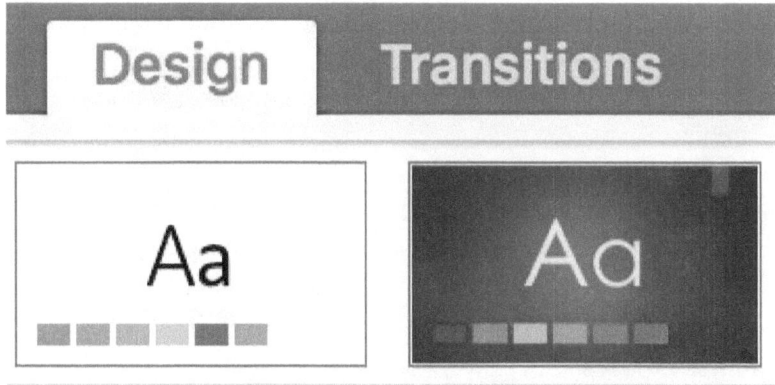

Another option to manage coloured background is called **'design'** and found on the icon bar. The design frames are tempting to use. Each theme has a pattern design and allows colour combinations to be added using one of the palletes. Stick to ONE colour theme throughout. Think of your audience rather than use a design for the sake of a personal attraction to variation.

It is perfectly permissible to insert a logo to one side of any slide, especially if you represent a firm or business. Try to make the logo small and discreet. Smaller text might be permitted in cases where a business name is required or reference to information which should be readable. Again, coming back to size. Small letters otherwise will not be visible from the back of the room. Imagery helps concentrate your audiences' attention where you want it. If you desire to consider another option, you can work through the cascade presented until you find what you want. The bar highlighted after selecting design allows you to change all of your slides with one click of a button. Colour schemes and patterns can be changed using the previous menus.

Next I have used one of the templates as part of the border edge design. Here is an example using a black background from the design template with a border feature made up of bubbles

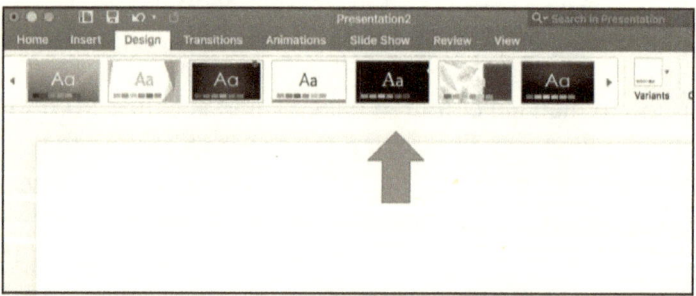

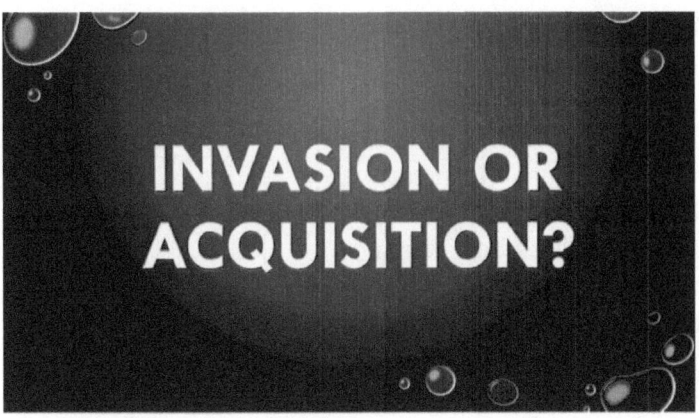

Always keep your slides simple although by all means experiment when confident. Before we complete this section I will introduce a little more about design of images before finally dealing with image transfer. Here is a summary of colour and text;

Text colours found to work well

White background and black text or black background with white text (best)
Blue (light) background with white or yellow text - good
Black background and a white border works well around edges of images
Yellow background blue or black text, or pale red can work but not best.
Contrasts can also be helpful as graduated colours.
Use images to achieve the maximum size so no edges if possible.
No background colour is required with full bleed picture images.

Manipulating Images

Tilting the image at an angle

First click on the picture that you have imported. A border is visible at each corner where the edge has white blocks. This was shown earlier where crop and sizing grab handles manipulated the slide image. Another way to move an image is via a rotating tool that exists on most boxes and shapes. A 360° movement can be achieved.

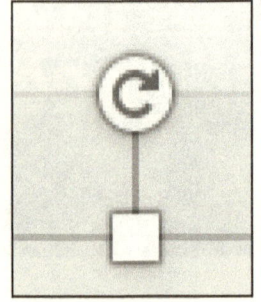

The C-shaped arrow points clockwise from the uppermost box with a vertical line. Place the mouse cursor over the circle and rotate the image either left or right so the image leans at an angle. Angled images can create a certain impression of asymmetry. Book covers for example can be pasted into the slide and tilted. See the left hand image over the page.

Overlapping images

Another useful feature when combining two or more images is the overlap feature. Import your images first and size them up by either taking the edge of each and increasing or decreasing the area. You can also put a measurable value in using the selection menu once back in '**Picture Format**'. Page 148.

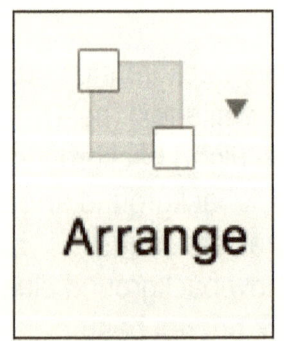

The height and width are given in metric (cm). **Bring Forward** or **Send Backward** headings appear and allows the image to overlap the way you wish. Page 164.

Ensure that you check the slide when expanded that this is the view you require for the audience and that the overlap should not obscure any feature you want. Rearrange the images to make sure each one does what is required in that sequence.

Once in **'picture format'** which is achieved by clicking on a slide, the drop down menu appears and contains the key items to bring the image forward or sent it backwards. Once this has been acted upon the photos overlap the other way as shown in the illustration. Because there are so many other options it is not appropriate to go into every permutation further. Some of the other methods can be experimented with as confidence grows. There is so much more to learn about images but one last topic worth talking about impacts on the speaker big-time! This is transferring data, backing it up and not turning up with the draft version instead of the beautifully honed PowerPoint programme you have sweated over.

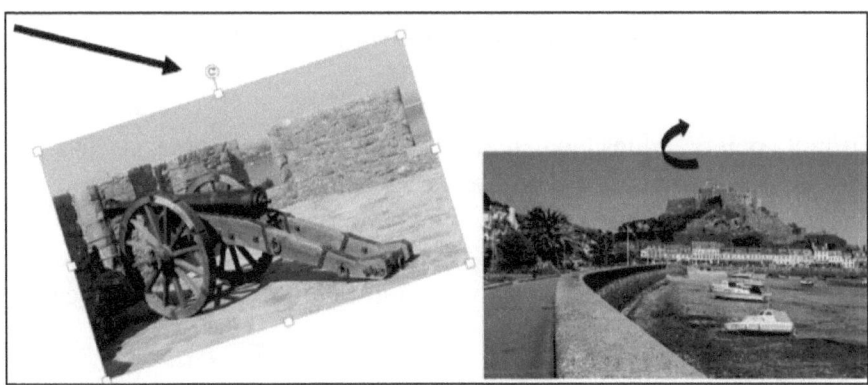

You can see that the top pictures have been repositioned at an **angle** while the bottom pictures have been **overlapped**.

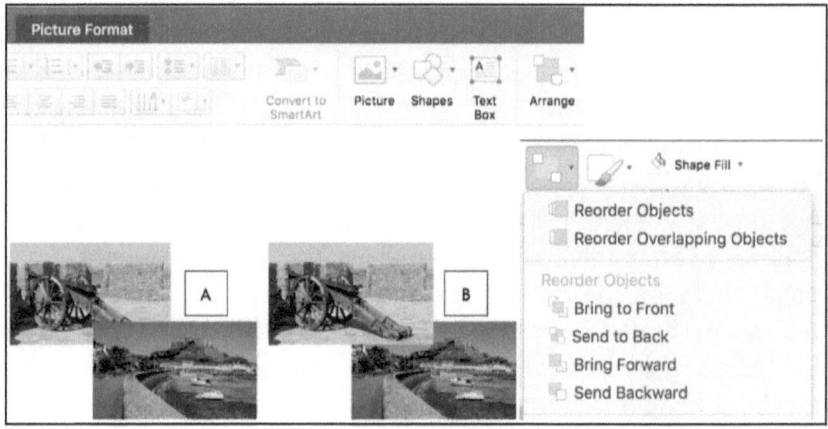

Political Correctness

You can use images from a digital camera or taken from the Internet. I used to think it was fun to put pictures of my children up and a practice in vogue several years ago. The idea behind the speaker having another life style appealed but of course there was a little hubris involved showcasing wealth for some, as background told another story.

Current society values have altered and showy off pictures are in poor taste and pictures of children (*even your own*) are subject to disapproval in a public setting. With data protection climbing another notch in May 2018, what we use and even say is under close scrutiny and permission plays a very significant role in what we can use.

The internet is valuable as a library for images and there are sites to download free material and sites you pay to download to overcome copyright. It perhaps should go without saying again, facial pictures need permission and written permission explaining how the picture will be used. The law changes constantly and the media have been at the centre of some of the controversy in recent years and so only use material covered by consent or license.

23 - Backing up

'A PICTURE IS WORTH A THOUSAND WORDS BUT IT TAKES 3,000
TIMES THE DISK SPACE.' - AUTHOR UNKNOWN

It is important to 'back up' your hard work in order not to lose it
accidentally. Reducing an accident can be achieved as we have
explained earlier by using a *memory stick*, also known as a USB
(Universal Serial Bus) flash drive, or better still, use an external
drive. We need to consider storage, back-up and portable data

Data

While this section is more technical it is important to be aware of
problems caused by inadequate computer speeds and data storage. I
have delved into format and data size briefly in this next section. For
those with an interest, the smallest data is called Bits of which there
are 8000 bits to a Byte or B. It then goes up in thousands so 1000B =
1kB (Kilobyte), 1000 kB = 1MB (Megabyte), 1000MB = 1 Gigabyte
or GB. 1000 GB = 1 Terabyte. Beyond this there are more sizes but
they do not concern us at this stage. All computers are priced on the
basis of the capacity of their hard drives. That's the internal storage
part. They are also priced on the speed that data can be computed.
We should turn our attention to external methods of storage because
attending some venues will require transfer of data from your
computer hard drive to another hard drive or source before the talk;
more so at large conferences with good technical (I.T) support.

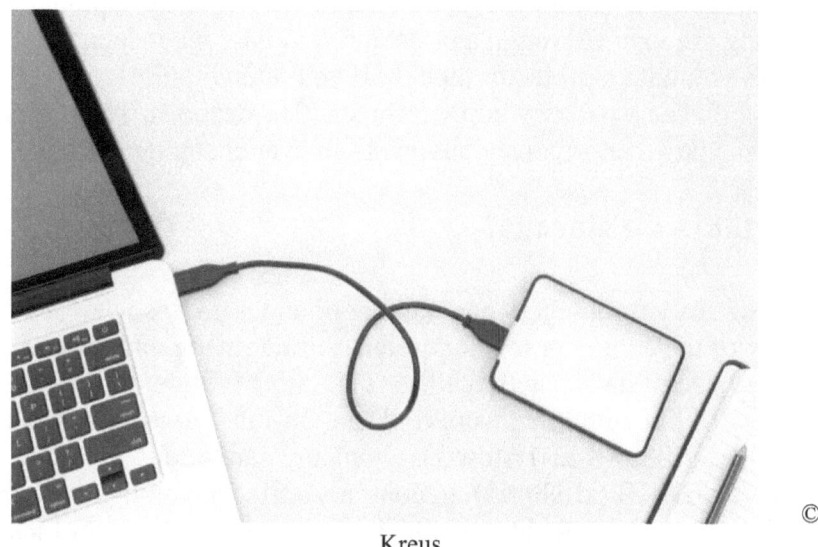

Kreus

It is custom and practice to take along a USB stick (invented in 1999). Portable external drives for data store larger capacities than the memory sticks[27]. Small capacity USB 'sticks' or flash drives are cheaper and are useful for keeping limited data in case material is lost. These memory flash drives can become corrupted, and then no longer readable. 1-8GB (gigabyte) drives are relatively inexpensive and can easily cope with most PowerPoint programmes even with high quality images. Larger capacity external drives are better for storing mass material off site. The storage called Cloud ideally is supposed to be safer still. Data is stored remotely and accessed only with internet connection if you are using another computer. A provider manages the cloud system. There are a number of cloud systems which provide some free data storage in GB (gigabytes). Once the limit has been reached you then pay for additional storage. The advantage? If your computer crashes or 'dies' you can access that same data using your access password.

---

[27] I use an external drive with 2 Terabytes. This has plenty of room on for my work as a back up but even these can become corrupted so consider a cloud system as well.

When attending small meetings, you may need your own laptop for projecting the image through a projector. It is vital the meeting provides you with a projector though. If you intend to do a lot of speaking it is best to buy your own for smaller meetings. The prices have come down enormously but this is an ever changing market.

What takes up storage?

As the size of your imagery and number of slides grow so the capacity of the computer memory reduces. Images are hungry for data. The size of data usually will start in units of kilobyte (KB). A simple word file with three words - 'Data-On-File', uses 22 KB. If a whole page (1081 words) is used without any paragraphs, it would increase to 168KB (kilobytes). In contrast, a file containing text might be relatively low but it would depend upon the amount of text and images used.

Artwork known as Clipart, diagrams and shapes use lower data while photographs, at best resolution, will increase the data storage enormously. A recent PowerPoint package I used took up not KB but 60MB, (megabytes).

Transfer of data

Data capacity impacts on the ability to transfer data. Copying across or sending data by the internet becomes slower, although dependent on the speed of the server you use. If your server is slow as in some rural locations, you can wait a long time to upload a large file. Speeds are measured in megabits per sec (Mbps). In the UK a 2019 post from comparethemarket.com ran...

A good broadband speed for streaming is at least 1.5 megabits per second (Mbps) for TV services such as BBC iPlayer for standard streaming, or 2.8Mbps for HD quality.

> If it's Ultra HD you're after, you typically need at least 15Mbps for YouTube, while it's 25Mbps for Netflix or Amazon Prime Video.

As far as computers are concerned they will run at lower speeds with the internet but current speeds of 60 Mbps upwards are becoming the standard and superfast broadband speeds are being offered at 300 Mbps for 2020. In 2018-19 the UK (average of 22.37 Mbps) was 34th in the league of broadband for 207 countries. Taiwan ranked at the top and Yemen at the bottom

However we note that the average UK speed of 22.37Mbps (Megabits per second) is well below the 54.2Mbps recorded by Ofcom's 2019 fixed line broadband speeds report

Mark Jackson 2019[28]

On standard laptops with a modest hard drive full of data, the speed of loading up PowerPoint will change depending upon the computer specification. If you use a memory stick this is fine, but larger data on a stick will mean slower transfer loading and delivery. PowerPoint stored within the laptop hard drive is faster for opening PowerPoint.

Zip filing
If you need to move large data to another site, there are currently two ways to do this. By compressing digital data, data is squeezed into a smaller size.

---

[28] Mark Jackson is a professional technology writer, IT consultant and computer engineer (UK)

A file capacity of 85.2 MB was squeezed to 72.2MB. This is called Zip filing. This can make a file 15-16% smaller. You can purchase more speed and capacity if sending large data with a server but then it just means you are paying out more money on IT and we want to save money, more so if this is just a hobby.

Wetransfer
My server allows me up to 25MB of data only before the attachments (paper clip icon) refuse to send. Wetransfer allows data over 25MB and at the time of writing this is the current way to send large data. Wetransfer is free but watch out there are purchasable formats from Wetransfer and it is easy to click and start a contract.

YouTube
You may wish to incorporate video. This facility has now been digitised as analogue video recorders in VHS are no longer the unit of recording. Digital video may be large, depending upon the length of the film. Unless you are competent at using video embedded into your PowerPoint I would suggest delaying the experience until you are more seasoned. Downloading YouTube may be easier but you have to come out of PowerPoint and go onto the internet during your presentation as well as having good access speed to the internet. Nonetheless it works well and is a useful method to break up talks and reduce attention lapses.[29]

---

[29] The material is provided for guidance only. The information will change within a short period but it does provide an idea around data size and how it can frustrate the PowerPoint user when planning and designing talks.

24 – The Big Recap: Common Rules and Mistakes.

When starting out, keep slides simple. Your **voice** is your most important asset followed by quality **images**. **Text** plays the least important part within your slide deck.

Plan – Purpose – Presentation = Performance

Plan
1. Keep each slide to one point rather than mixing different ideas and themes.
2. Allow yourself plenty of preparation time.
3. Allow time to practice your talk. You will need several run throughs.
4. Build a simple deck with words as your planner and images as your story board.
5. Don't over design your introduction or header slide until you have content. Then refine this at the end.
6. Prepare to edit heavily. This is normal.
7. Once you have your content ensure this fits into the time allocated and do not try and use everything.
8. Colours: Pale background, darker text is best
9. Always back up your slide deck. Do this frequently.
10. Use images that do not pixelate or degrade when expanded.
11. Limit transitions and animations to only those essential slides.
12. Ensure permission or license pictures and artwork if not your own.
13. A blank slide from the office theme (PowerPoint) is more flexible to work with than from a template.

Purpose

1. Be clear WHY you are giving the talk.
2. A talk should inform, entertain and engage all audiences.
3. One theme, three relevant points is often best when starting out; write these out first to keep on track.
4. Try to tell a story starting with a good anecdote or case history associated with the subject.
5. A talk has a start (hook), middle (main content) and an end (draw together) to remind audience of key content themes.

Presentation

1. Don't learn your script, learn the order.
2. Check your slide deck before and ensure any transitions and animations work on different equipment.
3. Images should fit narrative and re-inforce the point to aid communication.
4. Only use images that have value and do not repeat your spoken words on the slide.
5. Use an image instead of text wherever possible.
6. Quality of images is important. Use the whole frame unless making a compound slide of text/image. Bleed edges to ensure best fit.
7. Avoid reading slides, make headings on cue cards.
8. Text should be minimal. Five words per line and five lines are optimal. Less or none is better.
9. The back of the room must be able to see your text. Ensure the font size is appropriate.
10. Only use text to enforce a theme or point.
11. If text is on more than one line, animate the list after speaking to that point.
12. If you write text below in the notes section take care if the slide deck is shared.
13. Keep to the same font designs and colour schemes throughout.
14. Use no more than two font designs.

15. Advise your audience if they need to take notes and make time allowance.
16. Use handouts but give these out afterwards unless they are so brief as to guide the audience through your talk with a view to aiding notes.

Quick check for your order

- Do you have too little or too much material?
- Does the start of the talk lead to the main content?
- Does the main section, the content and delivery have a logical flow?

If you have found this book useful please try *Projecting Your Image* which goes into more detail about planning, purpose and presenting.

25 - Author's note

I hope this book supports you in the role of a speaker although this is far from complete as it concentrates on the technical side of PowerPoint in the main. There is a great deal more about how to speak and so for this I recommend looking at my main text on public speaking from conference centres to village halls.

I began my career with little emphasis on the need to speak, although as a professional educationalist this changed with the need to take classes. While most of my writing comes from personal experience I have dipped into a number of sources which I have cited under references and bibliography.

When I found sources that agreed with my own interpretation of public speaking this gave me the confidence to publish my own thoughts. The sources I have named have been successful in their own fields. I am grateful for their written words. All have the same passion which is to embrace an audience, and apply their skills in communication to help us recognise the importance of providing a good talk after being invited to speak.

PowerPoint software will undoubtedly optimise your range in wonderful ways to wow your audience. Some of my tips and ideas committed to print may make you wiser, not because they are mine alone, but remember that there is a conviction that PowerPoint can damage your health.

Don't become a victim!

26 - Authors cited in this book

Eric Bergman is a Canadian media training consultant. His focus on not relying on PowerPoint caught my attention as I conceived this book. I felt it was a duty to provide a balanced side to the subject of using PowerPoint as a medium for delivery. His book *5 Steps to Conquer 'Death by PowerPoint'. Changing the World One Conversation at a Time*, published in 2012 by Petticoat Press.

Chris Davidson is a Managing Director of Active Presence based in the UK and provides support on the subject of presentation skills. A major key aim is in sales technique and media communication. His book *Winning Techniques for Public Speaking and Presenting. How to Influence People with Social Communication Skills* was an internal publication from Active Presence and e-book produced in 2017.

Joanna Penn also mentioned in my book, has tremendous energy. She writes about writing and produces fiction. I have heard her talk and although she calls herself an introvert, her passion overrides any sense of being unable to speak publicly. *Her book Public Speaking for Authors, Creatives and other Introverts* comes as an e-book and printed book published by The Creative Penn Ltd, 2014.

Akash Karia has taken time to review talks by a number of international speakers based on the concept of the TED talk. This is an easy read guide to slide design and covers some useful tips behind slide design. It fits in well with others I have referenced in my book on Thinking as we build our talk. His book *How to design TED worthy presentation slides* is favourable priced and better purchased as a book than e-book.

About the Author

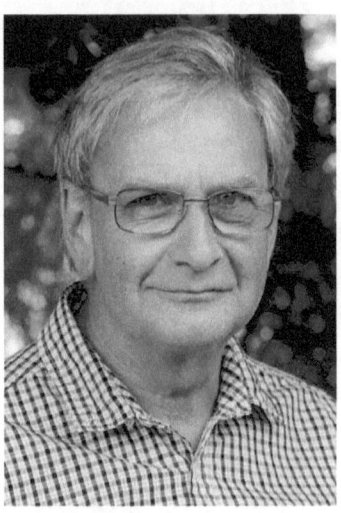

David has developed a strong interest in education, communication and public speaking over a 40-year career. He worked was Deputy Head and senior lecturer at Nene College of a Department of Podiatry, (now the University of Northampton) for 10 years and has been a visiting lecturer and course organiser at other universities. He has travelled worldwide to counties including Finland, New Zealand, South Africa, Israel, Ireland and the USA.

He decided to tackle public speaking because he was frustrated by the common mistakes he saw when people made speeches and presentations at the expense of overplaying PowerPoint. In his parallel book, *Projecting Your Image*, he reflects on his own mistakes. While the narrative is largely autobiographical it is intended to be as critical of his own failings as of others'.

David R Tollafield

Index

Foot Health Journey Books
from the same author

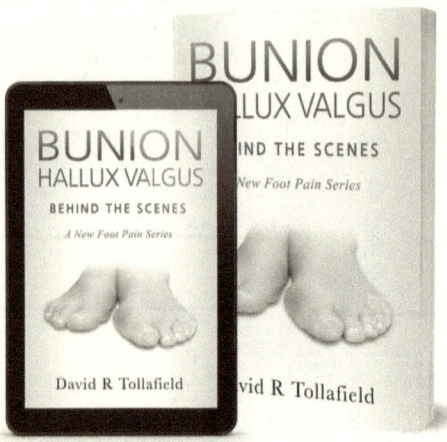

…I really wish a comprehensive book like this had been available prior to my first surgery…This 'warts and all' approach provides some very honest, frank and practical information and certainly would have prepared me for what lay ahead. - *J. Homer, Patient*

… I had to scratch around the internet looking at blogs, which mainly were American. In fact, had I read your book I may well have saved myself some money. Your book is extremely well written and I would highly recommend anyone considering surgery to read this first. There was more post-op information than anything that I could find! - *N. Harvey, Patient*

Foot Health Journey Books
from the same author

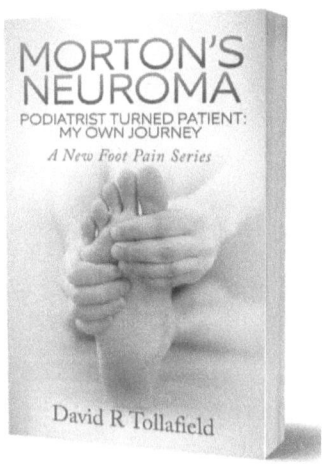

...Very easy to understand ... I would have found it helpful to have something like this as I was on google and wanted as much information as possible prior to surgery. -
Mrs Jenny Norton, Patient

...there is nothing like experiencing the symptoms and results of intervention for one self. This is why this book is so unique. -   **Mr Trevor Prior (consultant)**

...this book is very accessible and easily understandable by the lay reader/patient (due to its clear, simple and concise language) without losing any of its medical scientific value... -   **Dr Marius Vintella**